ADOLESCENT PARENTHOOD

ADOLESCENT PARENTHOOD

adolescent parenthood

Edited by
Max Sugar, M.D.

Clinical Professor of Psychiatry
Louisiana State University Medical Center
New Orleans, Louisiana

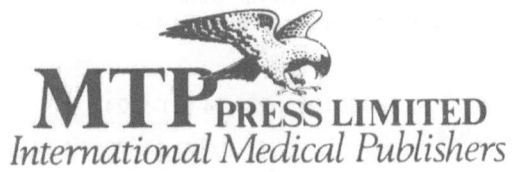
MTP **PRESS LIMITED**
International Medical Publishers

Published in the UK and Europe by
MTP Press Limited
Falcon House
Lancaster, England

Published in the US by
SPECTRUM PUBLICATIONS, INC.
175-20 Wexford Terrace
Jamaica, NY 11432

ISBN-13: 978-94-011-5926-5   e-ISBN-13: 978-94-011-5924-1
DOI: 10.1007/978-94-011-5924-1

Contributors

Nicholas Anastasiow, Ph.D. ● Professor, Department of Special Education, Hunter College, New York, New York

Jo Ann B. Fineman, M.D. ● University of Arizona Health Sciences Center, Tucson, Arizona

Susan M. Fisher, M.D. ● Lecturer and Consultant, Department of Psychiatry, University of Chicago Pritzker School of Medicine, Chicago, Illinois

James M. Herzog, M.D. ● Assistant Professor of Psychiatry, Harvard University Medical School; Faculty Child and Adult Psychoanalysis, Boston Psychoanalytic Institute, Boston, Massachusetts

Theodora Ooms, M.S.W. ● Director, Family Impact Seminar, National Center for Family Studies, Catholic University of America, Washington, D.C.

Carlos Salguero, M.D., M.P.H. ● Hill Health Center, New Haven, Connecticut; Assistant Professor, Department of Psychiatry, Yale University, New Haven, Connecticut

Kathleen Rudd Scharf, Ph.D. ● Tucson, Arizona

Nancy Schlesinger, M.P.H. ● Assistant Analyst and Educator, Management Information Services, Norwalk Hospital, Norwalk, Connecticut

Moisy Shopper, M.D. ● Clinical Professor of Child Psychiatry, St. Louis University School of Medicine; Training and Supervising Analyst, St. Louis Psychoanalytic Institute, St. Louis, Missouri

Marguerite A. Smith, Ph.D. ● Retired from Department of Child Psychiatry, Boston University, Boston, Massachusetts

Peggy B. Smith, Ph.D. ● Assistant Professor, Department of Obstetrics/Gynecology, Baylor College of Medicine, Texas Medical Center, Houston, Texas

Patricia Meyer Spacks, Ph.D. ● Professor of Literature, Department of English, Yale University, New Haven, Connecticut

Max Sugar, M.D. ● Clinical Professor of Psychiatry, Louisiana State University Medical Center, New Orleans, Louisiana

Edilma Yearwood, R.N., M.A. ● Staff Nurse, Inpatient Child Psychiatry Unit, North Carolina Memorial Hospital, Chapel Hill, North Carolina

Foreword

The definition of the risks of adolescent childbearing has received considerable investigative attention during the last decade. We have gradually moved away from simplistically studying young maternal age as the sole determinant of biologic and psychosocial outcome, even though we recognize it is one of several factors which warrant consideration.

We now recognize that if adolescents receive adequate and consistent prenatal care, they and their infants should do nearly as well as adult women and their infants of similar backgrounds. Thus, the major morbidities for adolescent mothers, adolescent fathers, and their infants are psychosocial: lack of educational and vocational futures, failed marriages, and dependence on government aid for support.

The adequacy of the parenting of adolescent mothers and fathers and the long-term developmental and physical outcomes of their children are largely unstudied. This book, edited by Dr. Max Sugar, a recognized authority on adolescence, focuses on the important topic of adolescent parenthood.

The authors of this timely contribution approach the topic of adolescent parenthood in a unique fashion, utilizing a combination of several approaches: consideration of fictional characters in history, astute and carefully conceptualized clinical observations, reviews of the literature, and their own investigation. It will be through the use of such a creative approach that we shall define the important questions which should be addressed about adolescents as parents and the outcome for their children.

The uniqueness of studying three developing beings—the adolescent mother, the adolescent father, and their infant—and their interactions with each other should provide future investigators special and exciting challenges. We are indebted to this book's authors for initiating the consideration of adolescents as parents.

ELIZABETH R. McANARNEY, M.D.
George Washington Goler Associate Professor of Pediatrics
The University of Rochester Medical Center
Rochester, New York

Preface

It is our view that the adolescent parent does not live in isolation but is part of a continued and involved extended family, and social and cultural group. Some of the participants in this larger tableau may or may not be willing to be identified or openly involved. But they certainly are affected by, and affect, the young adolescent females and males who become mothers and fathers. These include the infants, bilateral maternal and paternal grandparents, aunts, and uncles, as well as siblings of the adolescent parents. From these are derived a host in the environment who are members of the helping professions aiming to shepherd the youngster through the pregnancy and early motherhood. These include people who provide funding for her, as well as pediatric, social, medical, dental, obstetric, nutritional, educational, and other services.

The book takes all of these into the purview of the adolescent parents and their children. It is divided into four sections that deal with the adolescent and extended family, the infant and its developmental risks, some current programs for adolescent parents, and the implications for programs.

The opening chapter provides a review of cultural contributions to considerations about adolescent pregnancy, types of motivation involved, and views of men and women. Although adolescent pregnancy is not a psychiatric diagnosis, at times it has almost routinely been inferred in our scientific twentieth century, while in the nineteenth century it was seen as immorality requiring punishment.

Two chapters deal with different aspects of the problem of decision-making related to the adolescent becoming sexually active or using contraceptives. These areas have been looked at in various ways without providing a suitable response to the fact that most adolescents currently know about contraceptive use and yet ignore it.

The dynamic aspects of the adolescent girl becoming pregnant and being mother are examined. Another chapter focuses on adolescent males and their line of development toward fatherhood. A chapter differentiates young black and Hispanic mothers on the basis of ethnic factors.

Risk factors are described for the young mothers and their infants. The chapters on programs cover some different theoretical and practical aspects. The legislative history of funding for adolescent pregnancy and motherhood, which is not quite an illustrious reflection on our society, makes interesting reading about governmental management of its funds for these young people. The chapter on the extended families of the young parents reflects some beginning understanding, involvement, and support of the youngster's family through their adolescence and becoming a suitable parent. Although the cures for its slow development, as well as for improved legislative funding, are yet to be found, the authors of this section make some very thought-provoking points.

Hopefully, the book will inform physicians in all specialties involved with adolescents and their infants: obstetricians, pediatricians, neonatologists, psychiatrists, along with nutritionists, dentists, social workers, educators, legislators, demographers, anthropologists, sociologists, and those in the helping professions who may be dealing with the grandparents. This area has only recently become of interest to psychiatrists, primarily as a result of the risk features for the infants of adolescent parents for proper physical and emotional development. From this we have learned of the difficulties of these adolescents' emotional development, especially the young adolescent mother who is further burdened by having to look after an infant when she is herself still a child with her own unfulfilled developmental needs.

While this book may provide some answers and clues, it raises issues which may promote a broader and more appropriate view of the situation of the adolescent parents, their baby, and their extended family, including the helping professions and governmental apparatus. Hopefully, these will lead to improved programs that may be applied in a thoughtful and constructive fashion to deal with the growth and developmental needs of these adolescents and their infants'; this may avoid arrests in development for these infants and their youthful parents.

Acknowledgements

I wish to express my gratitude to the many who were instrumental, encouraging and supportive in this project: my wife, Barbara, for her editorial help and forbearance; my children for their support and tolerance for time away from them; my secretary, Marion Stafford, M.S., for her sprightly good humor and consistent efforts; Carol A. Leal, M.D., Taghi Modarressi, M.D., and John B. Reinhart, M.D., who were sources of stimulation and enthusiasm.

Contents

ADOLESCENT PARENTHOOD

ADOLESCENT PARENTHOOD

Adolescents
and the Extended Family

1

The Wages of Sin: Adolescent Mothers in Nineteenth-Century Fiction

PATRICIA MEYER SPACKS

In nineteenth-century English novels, sin means sex; sex demands punishment; illegitimate children symbolize or constitute that punishment. The good girl gone wrong almost inevitably appears soon in loose-fitting gowns, an object of scorn to her neighbors. She may die in childbirth or her infant may die; she may reform through a life of selfless devotion to others; but in no case can she successfully marry or bear subsequent children after a teenage mistake. Often she inhabits the periphery of a fictional action, functioning not as central character but as a moral warning or moral opportunity for more important figures. Her career—sin to punishment—follows so predictable a course that she holds relatively little obvious fictional interest, constituting an edifying embellishment more often than an imaginative focus.

The moralistic emphasis of much nineteenth-century narrative may obscure for modern readers a subtler psychological dimension in accounts of teenage pregnancy and motherhood. Long before Freud, novelists glimpsed connections between a girl's experience of being mothered and her own relation to mothering. At some level they saw (though they often concealed) emotional as well as moral meanings in the forces that drove girls toward sex and maternity despite the powerful social sanctions they incurred. To imagine the fate and feelings of social outcasts sometimes enabled novelists to hint at their own inadmissible responses, particularly at aspects of the contemporary female condition. Four important English novels, two from early in the nineteenth century and two from the Victorian period, suggest a range of imaginative possibility. I will consider Jane Austen's *Sense And Sensibility* (1811), Sir Walter Scott's *The*

3

Heart of Mid Lothian (1818), George Eliot's *Adam Bede* (1857), and Elizabeth Gaskell's *Ruth* (1853), the only one of these works to make an adolescent sinner its central character.

AUSTIN'S TREATMENT OF SEX

One does not readily associate Jane Austen with sex. In the foreground of her decorous novels, no one thinks of such things. Elizabeth Bennett in *Pride and Prejudice* (Austen, 1813) firmly asserts that her love for Darcy originates in her admiration for his estate; the joke uneasily emphasizes her utter refusal to acknowledge physical attraction as a component of love or marriage. Money is more acceptable than sex as a motivating force, and concern with money energizes all of Austen's plots. Yet, in the background of several Austen novels lurk sexual threats. Elizabeth's younger sister Lydia, for example, falls prey to a seducer. External forces rescue her before she falls to utter degradation, but her story stands as a dark threat of alternatives to the life of prosperity and ease which Elizabeth attains. *Sense and Sensibility* provides a sexual fable involving none of the characters whose problems shape the main plot. Its events take place offstage, narrated by Colonel Brandon for, he says, the purpose of comforting his beloved. The story occupies only a few pages; many readers forget it entirely. But in fact it calls attention to serious issues that the novel's relatively light tone disguises.

Colonel Brandon tells the story at a dark point in Marianne's fortunes. *Sense and Sensibility* follows two sisters through their education about the proper balance of emotional and moral qualities. At the outset, Elinor, the elder, exemplifies a preponderance of "sense." Too discreet to acknowledge openly her love for an eligible young man, she suffers in silence when her family moves away from his neighborhood and he neglects them. Marianne, on the other hand, a devotee of "sensibility," *never* suffers in silence. Her hero, Willoughby, appears on the scene in time to carry her into the house when she sprains her ankle; from then on she displays her infatuation with him, an infatuation which seems lavishly reciprocated. The two conceal nothing of their romantic involvement and their lack of interest in more mundane mortals. Willoughby leaves, however, without actually proposing marriage, and in London Marianne discovers that he will shortly marry someone else. Instantly prostrated by grief, she makes no effort to control her feelings or her revelation of them. At this juncture, Colonel Brandon appears. A middle-aged man with unexplained sadness in his background, he loves Marianne without hope of return. He tells his story to Elinor with the intent of communicating it to Marianne. "My object—my wish—my sole wish in desiring it—I hope, I believe it is—is to be a means of giving comfort—no, I must not say comfort—not present comfort—but conviction, lasting conviction to your sister's mind" (Austen, p. 148). His hesitations alert the reader to his story's ambiguous meanings and to his ambiguous purpose in telling it.

The story itself belongs to the familiar genre of tales of seduction and betrayal. Its pattern of generational repetition, however, differentiates it from most narratives of the sort. The first Eliza, Colonel Brandon says, strongly resembled Marianne: "the same warmth of heart, the same eagerness of fancy and spirits" (p. 149). Orphaned from her infancy, she lived, in effect, as the colonel's sibling, under the guardianship of his father. The two early acknowledged their love for each other, but "At seventeen she was lost to me for ever," married against her will to the colonel's brother, for the sake of the father's financial machinations. As the lovers prepared to elope, a treacherous servant betrayed them, Colonel Brandon was banished, and Eliza confined until she consented to the unwanted marriage. The colonel accompanied his regiment to the East Indies; Eliza promptly embarked upon a life of sexual looseness, culminating two years after her marriage in divorce, an event of course far more remarkable in early nineteenth-century England than today. Upon his return to England after five years, Colonel Brandon found her ill and destitute, with a three-year-old daughter, another Eliza. The first Eliza died of consumption; the colonel accepted the guardianship of the daughter, placing her in school until she reached the age of fourteen, when he put her in the care of "a very respectable woman" (p. 151). At sixteen, she suddenly vanished. Eight months later, the colonel found her, seduced and abandoned by Willoughby, and pregnant. We are told nothing about the child she bears, except that mother and child live now "in the country" (p. 154).

The story itself does not entirely support Colonel Brandon's claim that he wishes only to reveal Willoughby's villainy in order to reconcile Marianne to her loss. Both in its structure and in the colonel's emphases while telling it, the tale concerns the two Elizas far more profoundly than it concerns Willoughby. The narrative's conclusion underlines the point. " 'Such,' said Colonel Brandon after a pause, 'has been the unhappy resemblance between the fate of mother and daughter! And so imperfectly have I discharged my trust!' " (p. 153). The colonel's previous reference to "resemblance" has established a connection between Marianne and the first Eliza: "there is a very strong resemblance between them as well in mind as person" (p. 149). The unhappy resemblance of mother's and daughter's fates may extend to Marianne, like them in personality, unless a fortunate intervention rescues her from herself.

What determines disastrous female fates? The interest of the Eliza narrative in *Sense and Sensibility* derives from the fact that Colonel Brandon implies one answer to this question and Austen implies quite another. From Colonel Brandon's point of view, women allow themselves to be seduced and end up with illegitimate babies because no man watches them with sufficient care. His comment about how imperfectly he has discharged his trust—the trust of caring for the second Eliza—itself suggests his belief in the primary efficacy of male guardianship, but he has made the point earlier, in relation to the first Eliza. His brother, Colonel Brandon observes, "had no regard for her; his pleasures were not what they ought to have been, and from the first he treated her unkindly." Given the nature of Mrs. Brandon's mind, "so young, so lively, so inexperienced," the result was inevitable. "Can we wonder that with such a husband to provoke inconstancy, and without a friend to advise or restrain her (for my father lived only a few months after their marriage, and I was with my regiment in the East Indies), she should fall? Had I remained in England, perhaps . . . (p. 150). Female minds being what they are, males must bear responsibility; a bad husband produces a bad wife. Only a male guardian or friend might save her. By implication, Colonel Brandon suggests that he might protect Marianne as no female can. The grandiosity of this view, articulated by modest and retiring Colonel Brandon, has a startling effect. It derives from a kind of collective male narcissism, a phenomenon which Austen consistently observes and quietly mocks.

The larger narrative of the novel suggests a far different, and more psychologically interesting, interpretation of the two-generation disaster. Like all the teenage mothers in the novels considered herein, both Elizas themselves lack mothers. For Eliza I, the principal caring relationship involves the pseudo-sibling whom she wishes to marry; deprived of him, she can form no constant bond. The illegitimate daughter, born to her at 18, "the offspring of her first guilty connection," provides her only steady human tie. "She loved the child, and had always kept it with her" (p. 151). That child, orphaned, also enters a situation providing little emotional sustenance; her guardian, who cares for her, cannot keep her with him, and she spends most of her early life in a school, duplicating her mother's course presumably because, like her mother, she finds her primary emotional needs unfulfilled.

Beneath the moralistic surface of the story, in other words, lies a fable of emotional deprivation and longing, a fable of female need. The "resemblance" between both Elizas and Marianne extends even to Elinor, going far deeper than the colonel perceives. *Sense and Sensibility*, darker in tone and implication than earlier generations of critics noticed, relates in painful detail the desperate attempts and desperate reconciliations of two young women seeking emotional satisfaction in a world which provides little. Elinor conceals her feelings and her needs; Marianne displays hers. Both make satisfactory marriages, but neither in fact gets much. Marianne settles in the end for Colonel Brandon, a depressed middle-aged man more than twice as old as she; Elinor finds her reward in Edward, whom she wanted all along, but the reader wonders why: he too is depressed and passive. Both, however, avoid seduction and early pregnancy. Neither fully understands the meaning of the colonel's story about the two Elizas, even when Willoughby elaborates Brandon's version of events by reporting the intensity of Eliza's emotional needs and demands and explaining that the power of her feelings, rather than any evil in him, generated her downfall. "Her affection for me deserved better treatment, and I often, with great self-reproach, recall the tenderness which, for a very short time, had the power of creating any return" (p. 234). As justification for Willoughby, such an explanation exerts little force: the male betrayer remains blameable. But as a way of underlining the perception that girls have babies not because of badness but because of longing for emotional sustenance, Willoughby's account works well. Dramatically unhappy female fates, the kind of tragedy relied on by moralizers for centuries, take on new meaning in the context Austen establishes for them. Young women who get pregnant dramatize the plight of all young women in a world that seldom supplies emotional sustenance. Elinor and Marianne have a mother of sorts—weak and foolish, but loving. Given such security, they can escape the dark destiny of those who reveal too openly what they want and need.

The necessity of concealment, particularly for women, supplies a strong subtheme of *Sense and Sensibility*, in which virtually everyone has and must preserve a secret, and the novelistic action consists largely in the unraveling of secrets. People get through the world by obscuring their natures. Pregnancy and childbirth, difficult to conceal, represent from one point of view failure in relation to the system: girls who give birth outside of marriage have shown too much, violated the rules. From another point of view, pregnancy in the unmarried girl indicts the system, pointing to society's failure to give young women what they need. Only mothers—even the "bad" mothers characteristic of Austen's plots—give significantly to daughers. Orphaned, the young girl quite probably falls.

SCOTT'S TREATMENT OF ADOLESCENT SEXUALITY

Effie Deans, in Scott's *The Heart of Mid Lothian*, gives birth before she is eighteen to a male child who disappears while she tosses in delirium after parturition. Her mother has died many years before, although she has a devoted elder sister who tries to take the mother's place. Her strict, pious father, David Deans, shows no understanding of her human reality, judging everyone by the abstract standards of his scriptural interpretations. Deprived of emotional outlet (the older sister, virtuous Jeanie, largely accepts in action the father's doctrines), Effie seeks pleasure and finds it in the person of a dashing outlaw, George Robertson, whose promises of marriage help to account for her succumbing to his blandishments. With or without marriage, she remains devoted to him, refusing to reveal any information which might incriminate or endanger him.

Effie's destiny, more complicated than that of either Eliza, suggests Scott's concentration on the problem of what such "sin" as this means and implies. Although Effie as a character generates relatively little interest in the novel, which concentrates rather on Jeanie's story, her action (the sexual sin, the pregnancy, and its consequences) shapes the entire fiction. The book's title alludes to the Edinburgh prison in which, at the novel's opening, Effie lies in a semistupor of grief, confusion, and guilt, confined for the murder of her infant. That infant, whom she has never seen, remains the object of her desperate love, although at times she believes that she has killed it. She remembers no murder and she knows that she would never knowingly have committed such a crime, but the woman who attended her at childbirth has told her that she destroyed the baby in a maniacal fevered state; she can offer no counterevidence. Tried and convicted for the crime, sentenced to death, Effie hardly knows what she feels. She knows that she wants to live, she knows that she loves her seducer and the child she bore him, but she cannot sort out what she has done or what she wants others to do for her.

The prison, the title suggests, exists at society's very center, providing its vital force. The need to punish such sin as Effie's dominates the social structure, which cannot allow sexual freedom to women. No evidence supports the case for infant-murder; Effie is presumed guilty because she successfully concealed her pregnancy and its aftermath from everyone but the child's father and his accomplices. Concealment, in other words, which Austen suggested as the vital protection for individual need, here becomes the crucial sin. If a girl violates the sexual mores of her society, she must suffer the appropriate shame; otherwise the possibility exists that sin may go unpunished, that sexual pleasure may have no devastating consequence—a possibility which would undermine the substructure of moralistic decorum intended to control private and public arrangements. To make the private as public as possible protects the existing state of things. Effie violates important standards in her continuing insistence on privacy, refusing to reveal her seducer's name; she sneaks away, once pardoned, to rejoin him in secrecy, living for the next ten or twelve years virtually without communication with her family or country.

On the other hand, even Effie acknowledges the importance of public opinion. We first encounter her in her cell; her seducer has led a prison-breaking raid which would enable her to escape. She refuses to accept the opportunity, muttering, "Better tyne life, since tint is gude fame" (Scott, p. 75): death must follow dishonor. But she has other values as well. If, like the Elizas, she reveals her longing for a mother in her longing for a child, she also expresses her desire for independence. Her earlier adolescent development has displayed her need for self-assertion, which Jeanie proves unable to check. "Her sister, with all the love and care of a mother, could not be supposed to possess the same authoritative influence; and that which she had hitherto exercised became gradually limited and diminished as Effie's advancing youth entitled her, in her own conceit at least, to the right of independence and free agency. With all the innocence and goodness of disposition, therefore, which we have described, the Lily of St. Leonard's possessed a little fund of self-conceit and obstinacy, and some warmth and irritability of temper, partly natural, perhaps, but certainly much increased by the unrestrained freedom of her childhood" (Scott p. 112). Jeanie worries about the desire for freedom which she perceives only as danger, but she does not know what to do about it. She understands that to curb her sister too severely, as her father would attempt to do if he recognized her tendencies toward unrestraint, would do more harm than good, since "Effie, in the head-strong wilfulness of youth, was likely to make what might be overstrained in her father's precepts an excuse to herself for neglecting them altogether" (Scott, p. 116).

Although Effie of course does not consciously desire pregnancy, she has three powerful emotional forces driving her toward it. The need for privacy develops into a need for something of her own. Reared as she has been in an atmosphere of relentless moral examination, her father ever alert to details of appearance and conduct which might testify to his children's deviation from his own impossible standards, Effie must resort to stratagem, to disguise and concealment, in order to preserve anything for herself alone. Growing up in a time when paternal authority remained unquestioned, and subject to an unusually tyrannical (although by no means malicious) father, she would have to escape from his sight, from his realm of knowledge, to escape his utter dominance. Her yearning for autonomy, her second powerful motive, takes the form of rebellion against her father and his standards, and drives her toward her own eccentric choice of mate, despite the abundance of neighborhood admirers of whom her father would have approved. It drives her further still: to producing the child which would definitely assert an aspect of autonomy, at least in fantasy—giving her authority over one other human being. Daughter of an undemonstrative father, Effie longs for love; this longing becomes a third motivation. "It was not either in the nature or habits of David Deans to seem a fond father; now was he often observed to experience, or at least to evince, that fulness of the heart which seeks to expand itself in tender expressions or caresses even to those who were dearest to him. On the contrary, he used to censure this as a degree of weakness in several of his neighbours" (Scott, p. 163). The expression of love, like the assertion of autonomy or privacy, from the point of view of the stern father constitutes a sin. Effie commits all these sins in one in her liaison with George Robertson. Giving birth to an infant, an infant whose potential existence remains unknown even to her family, even more definitely fulfills her central fantasies, giving her what she wants: privacy, autonomy, love.

Effie's own scanty utterances about her seduction and her motherhood emphasize only love. She justifies her relationship with the outlaw by her extraordinary devotion to him. "If I hadna loved as woman seldom loves, I hadna been within these wa's this day; and trow ye, that love sic as mine is lightly forgotten?—Na, na—ye may hew down the tree, but ye canna change its bend" (Scott, p. 224). More important, perhaps, she claims his equally profound love for her. "How can I help loving him, that loves me better than body and soul baith?" (Scott, p. 226). She also stresses her passion for the unknown child she has borne. "O my bairn! my bairn! the poor sackless innocent new-born wee ane—bone of my bone, and flesh of my flesh!—O man, if ye wad e'er deserve a portion in heaven, or a broken-hearted creature's blessing upon earth, tell me where they hae put my bairn—the sign of my shame, and the partner of my suffering!" (Scott, p. 224). And again: "I wad hae laid down my life just to see a blink of its ee!" (Scott, p. 226). The notion of the baby as partner of her suffering reveals with special sharpness the purpose the baby—the *idea* of the baby— serves for her. Given a child of her own, she need never be alone again, isolated under the surveillance of moralistic father and uncomfortably selfless sister. She sees the child as an extension and a confirmation of herself; her fantasy of the infant functions thus even when the actual baby has vanished.

For a man in the early nineteenth century to imagine in such complex detail the motivating forces behind a youthful illegitimate pregnancy represents an extraordinary achievement. By Scott's principles as well as David Deans's, Effie is of course a sinner. Her punishment duly occurs as the novel continues, but the punishment, like the crime, derives from the workings of human nature. For Scott as for Austen (although Scott is usually described as having relatively little interest in the details of realistic characterization), the question *why?* has overwhelming interest. *Why* does Effie Deans bear a child in the first place? *Why* does the remainder of her life assume a shape largely determined by that adolescent event?

Part of the answer to the second question derives from Scott's understanding of the laws of poetic justice, by which the punishment always fits the crime. Part of it seems to depend on his interest in the ways that human beings create their own punishments by twisting their lives to answer obscure psychic needs. Unlike Austen, Scott interests himself in the male as well as the female parent involved in Effie's youthful indiscretion. Her seducer, known to her as George Robertson, has grown up in a rural rectory, a clergyman's son with a mysterious propensity for violence and danger. He accounts for his tendency to crime by suggesting that he imbibed it with the milk of his criminal wet-nurse, but a more plausible explanation would emphasize his rebellion against his stern and upright father, who espouses a different theological doctrine from David Deans but has similar views about child-rearing. (George's mother, too, is dead). At any rate, George, at the time when Effie meets him, has left home and dedicated himself to adventure rather than gain. He apparently intends to keep his promise to marry Effie, but finds himself imprisoned at precisely the wrong moment and can only arrange for Effie's care by a woman who in fact wishes vengeance against him as the seducer of her own adolescent daughter, who has become psychotic as the result of *her* teenage pregnancy. This woman spirits away Effie's baby. George, escaped from the gallows, rescues Effie from her father's farm, marries her, and eventually reassumes his upper middle class place in the world. Effie now has wealth, social status, a devoted husband. He supervises her education and presents her as the daughter of a Scotch Jacobite family; her beauty, natural intelligence, and surviving naïveté make her the darling of London society. She leads a glamorous and carefree life. Nonetheless, she remains miserable, for reasons closely related to her original motivations in becoming pregnant. Expert at concealment, yearning for privacy as a girl, she spends her adult life dedicated to a concealment which becomes torture; she must hide who she is and who her husband is, denying the identity she has sought to affirm. Longing for the love of a baby, something of her own, someone to care for her, she finds herself unable to bear another living child. Wishing to declare her autonomy, she leads a life of absolute dependence on her husband: more than usual dependence because of the lie at the heart of her existence. Without him, she would have no place, banished from Scotland as a condition of her pardon, branded as a youthful profligate, with no claims of personal accomplishment corresponding to Jeanie's. As for her husband: he too longs for a child, but not all his money or all his efforts can find the lost child, and his wife proves unable to provide a successor. He wishes for adventure but lives in the stultifying precariousness of lies. He suffers increasingly dramatic bouts of depression, a burden for his wife as well as himself; finally, in an improbable but psychically appropriate episode, he dies at the hand of his own lost son, neither father nor son knowing the identity of the other.

Effie envies Jeanie, who, making no claims for herself, wanting nothing, devoting herself always to the needs of others, has achieved a happy marriage in her own station, three healthy children, a sufficiency of money, and the love and admiration of all who know her: a model of female achievement. Want nothing for yourself, the novel says, and all shall be added unto you. Want what your father says you should not have, you will end in misery no matter what the world provides you. The moral, in other words, derives from the most conventional and simplistic doctrines of nineteenth-century Christianity. Unlike *Sense and Sensibility*, in which the novel's structure and the events it relates illuminate the implications of the Eliza story, in itself a minor episode, *The Heart of Mid-Lothian* seems organized to obscure the implications of its sexual fable. Austen reveals at every level of her narrative the ways in which society fails to allow satisfaction of the emotional demands of individual women. Scott, on the other hand, withdraws from the implications of Effie's story into a comfortable unexamined morality. He depicts Effie as having legitimate needs—autonomy, privacy, love—and as driven by her family situation to socially illegitimate means for fulfilling them. But by making Jeanie his heroine, making her a woman with no acknowledged needs beyond her passion for serving others, he enforces a negative judgment of Effie: not just because she has sinned, but because she has *needed* to sin. Jeanie rescues her and denies her emotional authenticity by insisting that there is no need to need. Scott, her creator, in effect does the same thing. He invents an action which allows her to survive, but insists on the unredeemable nature of the sin of self-concern: for women the unforgivable sin.

ELIOT'S TREATMENT OF ADOLESCENT MOTHERHOOD

George Eliot thought so too. In *Adam Bede*, she creates the unforgettable character of Hetty Sorrel, a seventeen-year-old rural beauty utterly absorbed in herself and her fantasies. Unlike other adolescent mothers in fiction, Hetty shows no discernible wish for a baby, although everything in her conduct indicates the likelihood that she will soon have one, and little affection for the baby she has. She too lacks parents, brought up by her aunt and uncle, the Poysers, and expected to help in the dairy and to participate in the care of small children. She rather likes the dairy, which shows off her pretty arms, but the children bore her; she displays no responsive affection for them and manifests no concern when, for example, the three-year-old she has tended briefly disappears into presumable danger. Her aunt Poyser thinks her hard-hearted, and the reader must think so too, although Eliot's analysis of her personality makes such a term as "heard-harted" an inadequate description. Hetty provides a case study of intense adolescent narcissism, so overwhelming that it cuts her off from true humanity, in the narrator's view. Repeated descriptions and metaphors associate her with subhuman nature: puppies, kittens, butterflies, water-nixies, flowers. "Hetty's was a springtide beauty; it was the beauty of young frisking things, round-limbed, gambolling, circumventing you by a false air of innocence—the innocence of a young star-browed calf, for example, that, being inclined for a promenade out of bounds, leads you a severe steeplechase over hedge and ditch, and only comes to a stand in the middle of a bog" (Eliot, p. 70). The analogy adumbrates the novel's plot, insofar as it concerns Hetty: Adam Bede literally and metaphorically pursues her on a different route, until he finds her in the dreadful bog of her moral inadequacy.

Moral terms come more readily to mind than psychological ones as one contemplates Eliot's fiction, but *Adam Bede* offers a penetrating analysis of Hetty's psychology. The limitations of the girl's imagination both derive from and intensify her self-absorption. Her "little silly imagination" (Eliot, p. 84) cannot admit the kind of lover who would demand of her full adult responsiveness. She prefers her fantasies of a fine gentleman; she cannot react to others' sorrows or needs. "Young souls, in such pleasant delirium as hers, are as unsympathetic as butterflies sipping nectar; they are isolated from all appeals by a barrier of dreams—by invisible looks and impalpable arms" (Eliot, pp. 84–85). Arthur Donnithorne, the young aristocrat who seduces her, embodies her male counterpart, equally irresponsible, equally far from adulthood although he is approaching his 21st birthday. The metaphors for their coming together emphasize the lack of will and thought involved: "Such young unfurrowed souls roll to meet each other like two velvet peaches that touch softly and are at rest; they mingle as easily as two brooklets that ask for nothing but to entwine themselves and ripple with ever interlacing curves in the leafiest hiding-places" (Eliot, pp. 111-112). But since Hetty and Arthur are in fact not peaches or brooklets or children, such imagery has sinister connotations. "Poor things! It was a pity they were not in that golden age of childhood when they would have stood face to face, eyeing each other with timid liking, then given each other a little butterfly kiss, and toddled off to play together. Arthur would have gone home to his silk-curtained cot, and Hetty to her home-spun pillow, and both would have slept without dreams, and tomorrow would have been a life hardly conscious of a yesterday" (Eliot, p. 110). The question of *consciousness* has central importance here. Eliot, a poet of consequences, stresses the necessity to take responsibility for the outcomes of one's acts; such responsibility depends on consciousness. Neither Arthur nor Hetty accepts the burden of consciousness; neither achieves it until both have paid heavy costs of suffering. Tomorrow, for adults, must always be a reminder of yesterday; the effort to escape consequentiality can only meet disaster.

Hetty's unawareness temporarily intensifies her pleasure. She dreams of a happy future in terms impossibly vague. "There was no knowing what would come, since this strange entrancing delight had come. . . . Hetty had never read a novel; if she had ever seen one, I think the words would have been too hard for her; how then could she find a shape for her expectations? They were as formless as the sweet languid odours of the gardens at the Chase, which had floated past her as she walked by the gate" (Eliot, p. 114). Arthur similarly indulges himself by refusing to specify the implications of his conduct. Never having read a novel, never having attended to evidence of how the world outside herself proceeds, unable to formulate generalizations or to perceive the laws even of fictional plot, Hetty lacks resources to combat her own dreaminess. Her career follows the same course as Eliza's and Effie's. Arthur leaves her, with a letter telling her he loves her but can never marry her and had therefore best not see her again. He has no cruel intent—the letter tells her to call on him in any distress—but also no intention of taking responsibility for his actions. Hetty agrees to marry Adam, but soon discovers her pregnancy. She flees, with the idea of finding Arthur where he has gone with his regiment, in Windsor. In Windsor she discovers that the regiment has moved to Ireland. Unable to follow it there, unable to bring herself to commit suicide, unable to face the disgrace of revealing her pregnancy, she wanders until she gives birth in a friendly woman's home, then leaves with her infant in the night and kills the child by burying it under leaves. She commits the murder, she explains to Dinah, out of a passionate longing to return to home, to undo the consequences of her actions and make everything as it had been before. "I thought I should get rid of all my misery, and go back home, and never let 'em know why I ran away" (Eliot, p. 390). Her ambivalence about the baby deters her briefly: "I longed so for it . . . I longed so to be safe at home. I don't know how I felt about the baby. I seemed to hate it— it was like a heavy weight hanging round my neck; and yet its crying went through me, and I daredn't look at its little hands and face" (p. 391).

Unlike Eliza and Effie, Hetty has experienced relatively little obvious emotional deprivation. Her aunt, strict, but affectionate, treats her almost as a child of the family. No one forces her to marry where she does not choose; no one forbids her seeking appropriate pleasure. She feels, however, like an outsider in her uncle's family, always conscious of the fact that she does not belong, unable to attach herself to it. Indeed, she appears to lack capacity for attach- ment. Her love for Arthur is all fantasy; she does not, like Effie, declare her undying love once he leaves her. He functions for her as an adjunct to herself, a mode of increasing self-esteem. Her love for the baby never distinctly manifests itself; the remark about its little hands and face represents her closest approach to a statement of feeling about the infant. Nor does she perceive the baby as a potential source of love for her: she lacks capacity, too, for postponed gratifica- tion. Depicted as a more pathological personality than Eliza or Effie, Hetty remains always trapped within herself. Adam cannot believe it, cannot imagine such a thing. Even as he hears testimony in court about the birth of the infant and Hetty's flight with it, he interprets her actions in relation to a normal capacity for love. "Hetty could not be guilty of the crime—her heart must have clung to her baby—else why should she have taken it with her? She might have left it behind" (Eliot, p. 374). But the previous narration has offered abundant evidence that Hetty can feel little but desire for her own gratification. Even as she struggles in her distress to reach Arthur, she does not think of him as some- one she loves, only as someone who will take care of her. She has always been taken care of; she wants more of the same.

Unlike Scott or Austen, Eliot provides no explanation for Hetty's mother- hood which might encourage the reader to sympathize with her or to condone the moral lapse such maternity represents. Hetty, too, has her female needs, but the narrator perceives them as reprehensible, not properly to be indulged. (Eliot's well-known animus against physical beauty may help to account for her harshness about Hetty.) Scott's contrast between Effie's neediness and Jeanie's firm repression of all need gives the moral advantage to the selfless woman, but he leaves room for sympathy with the more self-concerned one. Eliot's contrast of Hetty with the saintly Methodist preacher Dinah (whom Adam Bede eventually marries) allows no comparable option. "Hetty answered with a dimpled smile, as if she did not quite know what had been said; and it made a strange contrast to see that sparkling self-engrossed loveliness looked at by Dinah's calm pitying face, with its open glance which told that her heart lived in no cherished secrets of its own, but in feelings which it longed to share with all the world" (Eliot, p. 119). Concealment implies self-absorption; Eliot understands the youthful narcissism which controls Hetty and depicts it with merciless clarity. She shows no comparable understanding of Dinah's psychology: the saint operates by moral rather than psychological laws, privileged. She gives up her preaching at the end in order to function as a wife; her nature resolutely subordinates itself and the novel reveals no costs of such subordination.

Despite her lack of sympathy for Hetty and her unquestioning acceptance of the superhuman ethical commitment represented by Dinah, however, Eliot, like the other novelists considered, demonstrates her awareness of realities elucidated for our own world by modern psychoanalysis. She understands the engulfing power of narcissism, its capacity to assimilate all experience into an undifferentiated adjunct to the self. She understands the consequences of lack of an early object tie: the kindness of Hetty's aunt cannot help the girl to form attachments. And she understands that such a girl as Hetty might unconsciously long (most of Hetty's experience, Eliot makes clear, takes place below the level of consciousness) for a narcissistic extension of herself in an infant, and that the child itself, so visibly *not* an extension of the self, would prove intolerable to her. If Eliot's imagination is harsher than that of her predecessors, it is also acutely and unsparingly realistic. Alone among English novelists, so far as I know, she could allow herself to entertain the possibility that a mother might not in any meaningful sense love her child. And she thinks about the possible explanations for such "unnaturalness": Hetty lacks the vital connection to her own mother; her sense of herself as an outsider in her uncle's family urges her inward; she has few resources of intellect, knowledge, or doctrine with which to resist her own selfishness. At the novel's end she avoids hanging but suffers transportation to America, an appropriate fate for one who has never felt that she belongs.

GASKELL'S TREATMENT OF TEENAGE MOTHERHOOD

Elizabeth Gaskell's *Ruth* occasioned moral controversy in Victorian England. Its central character not only survives a youthful indiscretion, she thrives as direct consequence of a lie—a lie originated by the clergyman who rescues her, but acceded in and enacted by Ruth herself. Moreover, the fallen girl grows into a moral heroine, her sin providing the means of her redemption: the illegitimate child transfigures its mother. Mrs. Gaskell and her defenders argued the Christian purpose of the fable; no one commented directly on the passionate rage against men embodied in the avowedly Christian heroine.

Ruth's mother survives until the girl reaches the age of twelve. A strong, loving woman, she keeps the family going despite the mysterious incompetence of her husband, a man for whom nothing works out right, a man incapable of effective action. After his wife's death, the father disintegrates, dying some three years later of nothing more specific than lack of will and purpose. An unconcerned guardian apprentices fifteen-year-old Ruth to a dressmaker, in whose establishment the girl finds little support, comfort, or love. After her consumptive friend Jenny leaves, compelled home by her illness, Ruth feels altogether isolated; she succumbs to the handsome young gentleman who offers attention and apparent concern.

Ruth's intense need to love links her with Charlotte Brontë's heroines. Unlike Eliot's Hetty, the gratified recipient of love and admiration, Ruth hardly allows herself to recognize admiration when she receives it. She mainly seeks someone to care for. When Jenny becomes ill, Ruth longs to nurse her; when she sees a child fall into icy water, she rushes futilely after him. If she cannot have a mother, she will be one; and soon enough her longing to replace the dead mother is literally fulfilled.

The handsome young man abandons her at the instigation of *his* mother. (Living mothers and surrogate mothers in the novel, unlike the saintly dead mother, embody the split-off "bad" parent.) Alone, desperately worried about the lover who has been ill (she has, of course, nursed him until his mother arrives), frantic with grief, unaware of her pregnancy, she is rescued by a clergy-man and his middle-aged, unmarried sister. When a doctor tells them and Ruth of her pregnancy, Ruth responds—taking it, Miss Benson comments, "just as if she had a right to have a baby"—"Oh, my God, I thank Thee! Oh, I will be so good!" (Gaskell, p. 117).

Unlike Effie and Hetty, Ruth indeed feels it her right to have a baby and to have it alone, as though by immaculate conception. The man, having fulfilled his necessary function, need only disappear. Ruth's superlative goodness (she becomes ever more saintly until she dies as a result of nursing her former lover, not for love but from pure charity) derives from her maternity. And despite the novel's explicit insistence on the sin and sadness of such motherhood, the narra-tive reveals ever more clearly that only *because* of the illegitimacy of her child does Ruth find such gratification through it. Her own father seemed more or less irrelevant by comparison with his more effectual wife; Ruth intensifies her mother's pattern by eliminating the man altogether. When he reappears, years later, she fears that he will deprive her of the child, an emotion which supersedes all others. By the conventions of her society she, as a "fallen woman," can never marry, so her illegitimate motherhood saves her permanently from the necessity of allying herself with a male. The novel thus organizes itself around an adolescent pregnancy understood as an instrument of dual salvation. Overtly, the narrative reports how Ruth makes herself "good" as a reuslt of her joy in, and obligation to, her child. Covertly, it reveals how she saves herself from the Victorian woman's customary subordination to a man and how she expresses, through a life of self-sacrifice and devotion, her anger at males.

The one "good" man in *Ruth* exemplifies, like the protagonist, traditional feminine virtues: a crippled clergyman, thus doubly impeded from orthodox masculinity. Only three other significant men inhabit the novel's world: Ruth's seducer, irresponsible in youth and equally lacking in moral substance when he grows into wealth and political prominence; Mr. Bradshaw, a wealthy nonconformist whose rigidity and lack of perception make him, too, cruel, and, like the seducer, an object of the narrator's contempt; and Mr. Farquhar, who briefly thinks himself in love with Ruth but lacks the courage to contemplate continuing his suit, once scandal touches her. All the "masculine" men, in other words, are moral weaklings. Every woman, with the possible exception of the shadowy Mrs. Bradshaw, demonstrates strength; if two females turn their force to bad purposes, even they have more to recommend them than the men. Regardless of their social positions, the women in this novel demonstrate their effective autonomy. Ruth herself achieves through her pregnancy—despite her unfailing orientation toward others—a degree of autonomy far beyond anything Effie Deans could even have imagined.

A series of dreams reported in the narrative suggests the psychic course of Ruth's life and the way the pregnancy shapes it. At the beginning, the positive image of the good mother dominates her sleeping and waking thoughts. Her first reported dream tries to recapture the childhood relation to the mother; she wakes from it weeping bitterly. "I thought I saw mama by the side of the bed, coming as she used to do, to see if I were asleep and comfortable; and when I tried to take hold of her, she went away and left me alone—I don't know where; so strange!" (Gaskell, p. 9). The next night she dreams of the man who will seduce her.

One figure flitted more than all the rest through her visions. He presented flower after flower to her in that baseless morning dream, which was all too quickly ended. The night before she had seen her dead mother in her sleep, and she wakened weeping. And now she dreamed of Mr. Bellingham, and smiled.

And yet, was this a more evil dream than the other? (Gaskell, p. 18)

The ambiguous formulation suggests—not, presumably, by conscious intent, this being a mid-nineteenth-century novel—that dwelling in the image of the dead mother may have as dangerous an effect on Ruth as dreaming of a man above her station. Certainly her obsession with her mother does not protect her:

it means, among other things, her reluctance to grow up. Mr. Bellingham finds "something bewitching in the union of the grace and loveliness of womanhood with the *naïveté*, simplicity, and innocence of an intelligent child" (Gaskell, pp. 32–33). In a sense, Ruth's dependency on the image of her mother guarantees her seduction: she has developed no vision of herself as a separate, responsible human being. (Such a sense of identity must wait until she herself becomes a mother.) As much as the dream of Mr. Bellingham giving her flowers, the girl's intense concentration on the figure of the nurturing mother foretells her fate. If the good mother leaves her to loneliness in the dream, that mother must be restored. How better than by identification?

After Bellingham abandons her, Ruth considers suicide. Mr. Benson, the crippled clergyman, invokes her obedience in her mother's name. "In your mother's name, whether she be dead or alive, I command you . . ." (Gaskell, p. 100). Ruth cannot resist such an appeal. Her subsequent dreams, however, do not concern her mother.

> She dreamt that the innocent baby that lay by her side in soft ruddy slumber, had started up into man's growth, and instead of the pure and noble being whom she had prayed to present as her child to "Our Father in heaven," he was a repetition of his father; and, like him, lured some maiden (who in her dream seemed strangely like herself, only more utterly sad and desolate even than she) into sin, and left her there to even a worse fate than that of suicide. For Ruth believed there was a worse. She dreamt she saw the girl, wandering, lost; and that she saw her own son in high places, prosperous—but with more than blood on his soul. She saw her son dragged down by the clinging girl into some pit of horrors into which she dared not look, but from whence his father's voice was heard, crying aloud, that in his day and generation he had not remembered the words of God, and that now he was "tormented in this flame" (Gaskell, p. 162).

Her child, like her seducer, belongs to that male species marked by moral weakness but also by sinister power over women. Ruth's anger and fear emerge clearly in her dream. Her waking fantasy of totally possessing and controlling her son in the dream reveals its dark underside: it derives from her terror of what she believes men to be when *not* controlled by good women. Victimized herself by feckless father and lover, she converts victimization to strength, yet she knows the surviving danger of maleness.

The last sequence of narrated dreams underlines the point. It occurs after Bellingham has reappeared in her life but before she has spoken with him alone. "In her dreams she saw Leonard borne away into some dim land, to which she could not follow. Sometimes he sat in a swiftly-moving carriage, at his father's side, and smiled on her as he passed by, as if going to promised pleasure. At another time he was struggling to return to her; stretching out his little arms, and crying to her for the help she could not give" (Gaskell, p. 288). Now she imagines her son as readily corruptible by his powerful father, and she imagines herself as powerless mother, powerless to "follow" into the land of males, powerless to protect. She deals with her fear and rage in her waking life by reiterated refusal of contact with her lover, who wishes to resume relations, and her celibate life becomes increasingly noble in its selflessness until her heroic death—a death unwittingly caused by a man, the fundamental source of danger. Ruth can relate comfortably to men crippled or sick, not to the healthy and aggressive; but a sick man can kill her.

The adolescent pregnancy in *Ruth*, then, expresses the full meaning of the character and her career. Not socially sanctioned, such a pregnancy provides Ruth the opportunity for solitary possession of a child, her own child, focus of all her power. It supplies her an opportunity to identify with, and thus to recapture, the dead, good mother. And it expresses her helplessness in the ambiguous state of adolescence, looking like a woman, feeling like a needy, passive child, readily betrayed by a dangerous male.

DISCUSSION

In one way or another, the themes of youthful pregnancy as an expression of need and of pregnancy as involved with desire for concealment (both socially induced and more fundamental) run through these four texts. Gaskell, who provides the fullest imaginative study, also demonstrates the most sympathetic understanding of the dilemmas an adolescent girl's pregnancy may express and attempt to resolve. Austen, with the sketchiest presentation, also reveals her comprehension of the longing for emotional sustenance hidden within such acts of social deviance. Scott comprehends the same truth, although he draws back from it, unwilling to confront completely the implications of his perception. Only Eliot refuses to grant much sympathy to the victim of emotional deprivation, understanding her Hetty as deprived certainly, but refusing even temporarily to condone the moral insufficiency implicit in the girl's utter self-absorption. All four novelists convey their awareness that sexual sin results from no simple "badness" and that moral terminology cannot adequately describe its genesis or its consequences.

But the novelists practice their own concealments which have allowed many readers to believe that the tales of pregnancy embodied in nineteenth-century fiction serve only didactic purposes. From Austen's scanty summary to Gaskell's elaborate investigation, these writers use their century's moral orthodoxies to disguise their own social and psychological concerns. Each tells a version of the same simple story—sin, shame, punishment—although the notion of "punishment" in Ruth is sufficiently subtle that it apparently eluded many early readers. Each affirms the same pieties: sex is sin, and so on. But each also discriminates the psychic dynamics of this crucial sin: those who can will see behind the pieties.

Adolescent pregnancy supplies for these novelists a kind of paradigm of the female condition, an expression of needs unfulfilled by society, of longings not acceptable in woman but forcing their way out. Even Eliot, who imagines the adolescent mother as controlled by pathology, perceives the pathos of Hetty's helpless yearning for the love and approval and security which a mother might have given her. These imagined motherless girls reveal the power and the danger not so much of female sexuality as of female feeling. They also provide pretexts for exposing the irresponsibility, self-indulgence, and arrogance permitted men in nineteenth-century society. Long before Thomas Hardy created *Tess of the D'Urbervilles*, novelists criticized the double standard; long before Freud, they investigated consequences of women's sexual repression.

SUMMARY

Four nineteenth-century English novels which appear to offer conventional stories of sexual sin and retribution in fact reveal subtle psychological perceptions of the dynamics of teenage motherhood. Jane Austen, in the tiny story of the two Elizas embedded in *Sense and Sensibility*, dramatizes the exigencies of female need for emotional sustenance through the tragic fates of mother and daughter, both parents of children born out of wedlock. Sir Walter Scott, in *The Heart of Mid-Lothian*, depicts adolescent pregnancy as the product of rebellion and self-assertion against parental restriction. George Eliot's *Adam Bede*, the darkest of these stories, tells of a girl whose narcissism drives her first to pregnancy, then to infant-murder. In *Ruth*, Elizabeth Gaskell explores the fate of a girl who identifies with her own mother through an illegitimate pregnancy and achieves her salvation by rearing the child. All four books emphasize the pressure of women's needs and the limitations of socially acceptable fulfillment for such needs.

REFERENCES

Austen, J. 1976. *Sense and Sensibility, The Complete Novels of Jane Austen,* Vol. I. New York: Random House. (First published 1811).

Austen, J. 1976. *Pride and Prejudice, The Complete Novels of Jane Austen,* Vol. I. New York: Random House. (First published 1813).

Eliot, G. n.d. *Adam Bede, Novels of George Eliot.* Vol. I. London: Blackwood. (First published 1857).

Gaskell, [E.]. 1906. *Ruth and Other Tales.* London: Smith, Elder. (First published 1853).

Scott, W. 1956. *The Heart of Mid-Lothian.* New York: Dutton. (First published 1818).

2

Adolescent Decision-Making Toward Motherhood

MAX SUGAR

It seems useful to separate the decision-making components on the path to adolescent motherhood from the beginning of sexual activity through the post-partal period.

Among the decisions involved are engaging in sexual intercourse, the use of contraception, pregnancy, abortion, adoption, early motherhood, marriage, unwed motherhood, and further pregnancies in adolescence. These are affected by the girl's relationship to her family of origin and have effects on the child raised by the young unwed mother, the girl's emotional development to adulthood, the girl's socioeconomic and academic development, and her family of origin.

CURRENT ASPECTS OF ADOLESCENT MOTHERHOOD

The United States has the highest rate of adolescent pregnancies of all industrialized nations, along with one of the highest infant mortality rates, which involves rural, urban, white, and nonwhite girls. In 1971, 26.3 percent of white teenage girls between 15 and 19 years of age had had premarital sex and about six percent became pregnant; however, in 1976, for this age range, 37.2 percent had intercourse and ten percent became pregnant. For black girls of similar age for these years, the figures for intercourse also increased, from 54.1 percent to 64.3 percent; however, the percentage of those who became pregnant remained at about 25 percent for both study years.

In 1976, the rate of illegitimate births among blacks was 50.3 percent—almost double that of 1965. This appears to be due to increased contraceptive use among married black women compared with the use by the single women. But the rate of illegitimacy among whites also almost doubled in the same period, going from four to 7.7 percent.

Abortions among white girls aged 15 to 19 increased from 33 percent in 1971 to 45 percent in 1976; for black girls at these ages, the figures rose from five to eight percent. The ratio of first pregnancies terminated by abortion among these girls, black and white, almost doubled: from 17.7 percent in 1971 to 30.6 percent in 1976. Within a year of giving birth, one of four girls is pregnant again. About 300,000 teenagers were having abortions annually before the recent restrictive HEW legislation was passed (Alan Guttmacher Institute, 1976; U.S. News & World Report, 1978).

In 1951, the teenage birth rate was 96/1,000; in 1974, it was 58/1,000, and 80 percent of these births were out of wedlock. Figures for abortion rates are still not entirely accurate although more are recorded now than a generation ago. At that time, most of the upper and middle class girls who did not have an abortion gave up the baby for adoption. At present, this group usually opts for an abortion, while lower or working class girls keep their babies in about 95 percent of cases (Fisher, 1978). The different maternity rates between the middle and lower class may be a reflection of the greater number of options available to those with better advantages, such as abortion, schooling, or job opportunities.

From one view this results in 11.7 billion dollars spent annually in federal, state, and local Aid to Families with Dependent Children (ADC); women who thus are dependent in their teens cost taxpayers about six million dollars per year in welfare funds.

However these facts smart, they are impersonal; each adolescent who begins coital activity early, becomes pregnant (or not), carries to term (or not), keeps her baby (or not), is a unique and separate individual with a specific personal history and family, dynamics, cognitive abilities, educational attainments, and talents. At each stage along the road from beginning sexual activity to motherhood there are some very specific and significant decisions to be made by each individual girl.

THE DECISION ABOUT CONTRACEPTION

The decision to become sexually active is a complex one. Those looking at it from only a social or economic viewpoint miss the multiple emotional tributaries and the contributions from the family, the antecedent personal development as well as the prior and current reality situations. Furstenberg (1976) noted that in the very strict families among the lower social class the girls were more likely to become sexually active earlier than in the more liberal or less rigid family. Early coital activity was also partly related inversely to the girl's educational ambitions.

Early sexual activity is rarely promiscuous and occurs most often in the context of repeated intense relationships (Kantner and Zelnick, 1972; Sorensen, 1973). Sexually active white girls had more partners than black girls of the same age, but 70 percent of white girls had only one partner (Kantner and Zelnick, 1972).

Psychological and sociological theories are at odds in explaining the low use of contraceptives. A study of nonpregnant mentally ill teenagers for factors in nonuse of contraception (Abernathy and Abernathy, 1974) indicated that high-risk girls, in contrast to virgins, more often had relationships with their fathers which excluded their mothers; they depended less on their mothers for sexual information, while the virgins expressed open dislike for their fathers. Gottschalk et al (1964) found no evidence of any undue psychiatric disorder before pregnancy in a group of pregnant and nonpregnant white and black girls.

Educational ambitions most accurately predicted the eventual successful practice of birth control by previously pregnant youngsters (Klerman and Jekel, 1973; Furstenberg, 1976).

As is well known, the hormonal levels and the regularity of ovulation and menses are not predictable or reliable in the first few years after menarche; thus, fertility rates are low in these years. But this may be used as part of a pattern to deny the possibility or the effects of sexual activity. "The pattern of frequent dating over a long period is eventually accompanied by sexual activity and few adolescents are able to remain sexually active for long before pregnancy occurs" (Furstenberg, 1976). Furstenberg (1976) found that the mother's estimate of the incidence of sexual activity of the nonpregnant teenage daughter was so low that it suggested that she (mother) had a stake in being misinformed, which released her from responsibility to prevent pregnancy. An example of extreme denial is the 15-year-old white middle class girl who saw her pediatrician with her mother about general malaise. A short while later she delivered a full-term infant in his office, with the girl and her mother claiming ignorance of the pregnancy.

Kantner and Zelnick (1973) noted that 25 percent of 13 to 15-year-old unwed girls had used contraception. Furstenberg (1976) found that only 6 percent of his study group were unable to identify any method of contraception. Fisher (1978) felt that 80 percent of teenaged girls had knowledge about contraception but did not apply it. Possibly much of the increased sexual activity may be a reflection of the current sexual freedom and better birth control methods. In 1976, 30 percent of sexually active teenagers used contraceptives—an increase of 12 percent from 1971.

A frequent finding in programs to aid the pregnant teenager is the conflict with the parents about the daughter's sexuality (Nadelson, 1974; Fisher, 1978) and the family plays a part in transmitting expectations about birth control. Parents may supply information, by which they reveal awareness of the daughter's coital activities. The adolescent is then allowed to acknowledge her own sexuality and hence may regard sex less as a spontaneous and uncontrollable act and more as an activity which is subject to planning and regulation (Furstenberg, 1976).

Hattie Williams (1978) noted from her personal experiences as a volunteer in a Chicago black ghetto that these girls lacked simple knowledge of physiology and adhered to fearful superstitions about contraceptive pills. One girl was unprotected against the rapacious young men in the building and allowed herself to be used by the boy who raped her since "you have to have one boy so he'll protect you from the others, or they'll run a train on you." But most black and white pregnant girls are not living in such an environment. Are parents negligent in this respect? Are the girl's needs to "go steady" also reflecting other needs such as loneliness, fears of fusion with mother, etc.?

In the Baltimore black ghetto (Furstenberg, 1976), brief sexual encounters often were unexpected and undesired; virtually none of these women had used birth control. In contrast, among the women who were still seeing the father of their child, a majority (69 percent) had used contraception if discussion of birth control had occurred in the home. When parental intervention was absent, only 22 percent had contraceptive experience before conceiving. To a great extent, the influence of the family depends on the nature of the couple's relationship.

The assessment of the adolescent mother is complicated by the fact that most studies are retrospective, without controls, and converge on—instead of separating—facets of some of the most complex and difficult emotional and developmental adaptations: adolescence, pregnancy, and parenthood with or without marriage.

Is the early onset of menarche (12.8 years) (Petersen, 1979) condensing the prepubescent and latency phase so much that early onset of coital activity and pregnancy are natural results? In this country and England, historically, the average age for first pregnancy until recent decades was in the early twenties (Wynne and Frader, 1979).

Some regard adolescent motherhood in whites as due to psychopathology and in nonwhites as due to sociological factors. Kinch et al (1969) felt that the majority of these youngsters are neither very disturbed nor promiscuous. The causes given for adolescent pregnancy vary from all or none of psychological, social, biological, and economic features. Most research on this is limited, faulty, or biased. Psychiatric studies are usually small, without controls, and deal with a patient population that is pregnant. Bonam (1963) theorized that pregnancy was an escape from conflict, especially with the mother, and that the patients had narcissistic character disorders. Khlentzos and Pagliaro (1965) considered the pregnancy as a means of meeting oral dependency needs. Barglow and associates (1968) found problems of passivity, dependency, and depression. Babikian and Goldman (1971) related acting out and a weak ego to the pregnant adolescent. The girl who has a character disorder, oral dependent problems, or other neurotic problems is quite different from the schizophrenic or the manic, pregnant or not. Pauker's (1971) longitudinal study stressed that there was no one personality or motivating causality model to explain all out-of-wedlock pregnancies.

Sarrel and Davis's (1966) assessment of the pregnant teenager was similar to that of Webb et al (1972): the teenager had a syndrome of failure—"failure to fulfill her adolescent functions, remain in school, limit her family, establish stable values, be self-supporting and have healthy infants."

Schaffer and Pine (1972) found a regularly recurring theme of conflict in the pregnant girl about mothering and being mothered, as well as gross denial. Nadelson (1974) stressed the factor of denial in relation to the largest number of requests for late abortions arising in adolescents. She also noted that pregnancy in an adolescent may be a way to announce her adulthood, that pregnancy may be a response to a loss, often of a parent. Coddington (1979) found that in the preceding year in a group of pregnant adolescents, 54 percent had a death in their family in contrast to 23 percent among controls, and 50 percent had a family illness in contrast to 31 percent of controls.

Among those of low socioeconomic status (SES), Sugar (1979) found that in their pregnancies 56 percent of adolescents compared with 35 percent of adults had serious crises. A large number of these youngsters had a symbiotic tie with their own mothers and conflicts at a preoedipal and oedipal level (Sugar, 1979). "Pregnancy in an adolescent may be an unconscious effort to effect a separation; an attempt to make up for the loss of the infantile objects; a substitution and avoidance of early separation-individuation conflicts; or an accident to avoid regression" (Sugar, 1979). Cutright (1976) observed that decades of study have provided no comprehensive psychopathologic theory of illegitimacy. However, it is possible that middle class girls have been observed in considerable detail psychiatrically, whereas the lower class girl has instead been studied largely only sociologically or in obstetric clinics.

The sociological idea that a culture of poverty promotes premarital pregnancy has been seriously questioned by Furstenberg (1976). But his post partal observations about feelings during the pregnancy raise issues about methodology. In addition, it has been noted that as a result of being snowbound (for example, Boston, 1977–1978), the pregnancy rate goes up; it would seem logical to assume that the high unemployment rate of adolescents (especially of black adolescents) would affect teenage pregnancy rates. Schlackman (1966) believed that the association between poverty and early pregnancy was due to problems of access to contraceptives. Johnson (1974) correlated poverty with increased chances of adolescent pregnancy and pregnancy with increased chances of continuing poverty.

Plionis (1975) noted that the multiple theories of causality result from a lack of clarity in defining the problem and that this contributes to program design difficulties.

Vincent (1961) stated that most of the data about unwed mothers "may tell us less about factors contributing to illegitimacy than about the clientele of given charity institutions, social agencies, out-patient clinics, and physicians in private practice."

Among a number of borderline adolescents, I have noticed a pattern of symbiotic relatedness between mother and daughter, with such intense clinging that they go "barhopping" together or the girl goes out with mother's best female friend and they have an open rivalrous relationship over the teenager's boyfriends. In several instances, this situation has been a factor in the girl not using contraception and consequently becoming pregnant. Using denial as her defense, she feels she can't get pregnant, since the mother or the mother's substitute is there to protect her. What appears to be oedipal is really oral dependency in these cases, with little separation-individuation.

TERMINATE OR CONTINUE THE PREGNANCY?

After discovering her pregnancy, the next level of decision-making for the girl is whether to abort or continue her pregnancy. Before the 1973 Supreme Court decision, most therapeutic abortions were based on psychiatric indications. From then until the recent new law limiting some abortions there was a marked drop in the psychiatric need and requests made for diagnoses.

Frequently, abortion has been recommended by the physician and/or family without consulting the girl. Probably a similar percentage of girls decide on and obtain an abortion on their own to avoid being told what to do.

The selection of counsellors to aid the girl and her family to understand their situation, conflicts, possible choices, and services available to them is a crucial first step in a thoughtful, considered approach. The counsellor may then become the most vital and continued link in a support system, helping the girl arrive at her own decision while maintaining a neutral objective position. Counselling should be with the same person before and after abortion; it should provide support, information, and education as well as focus on the girl's motivation, ambivalence, ability to tolerate stress, ego strengths, and preabortion anxiety (Nadelson, 1974).

Nadelson (1974) found the presence of a successful maternal figure and the peer group fundamental to their program. The recidivists and the late abortion seekers were girls with special problems needing especially sensitive handling.

Recidivism in illegitimacy is usually associated with socioeconomic status and race. Among unwed mothers in Vincent's study (1961), 62 percent of county hospital blacks and 23 percent of county hospital whites were recidivists, compared with ten and seven percent of blacks and whites, respectively, in private practice and maternity homes.

Very aggressive pressures have surfaced recently to sway decisions against abortion; these have a disturbing effect on many girls' planning. Thus, a private decision has now become a matter for public forums on television and in other media, adding to the strain of the girl's decision-making.

The decision to carry through to term is often ambivalently based on hopes of a marriage; or, it may be in defiance of the parents' wishes despite the best of programs. The girl in the deprived group studied by Barglow et al (1968) appeared better adjusted at mid-term; however, in most cases resentment and depression followed the infants' birth. Gabrielson et al (1970) found that 13 percent of their study girls who had delivered before age 17 had attempted suicide. Furstenberg (1976) found retrospective unhappiness about having a baby in 80 percent of the single mothers. Only 20 percent of his group were married one year after delivery; of these, 79 percent were happy about the pregnancy. Over 60 percent of premarital conceptions (therefore not limited to teens) in one survey resulted in marriage (Cutright, 1976). But teenage marriages are problem-filled, as will be detailed further.

BE A MOTHER OR GIVE UP THE BABY?

If the girl decides to continue with the pregnancy to term, she has to consider keeping the baby or giving it up for adoption. This decision is complex and has many contributory channels which include the girl's psyche and conflict with her parents, the parents, the girl's wish for further education and a career, attitudes of rejection or acceptance by the culture and neighborhood, the socio-economics and options available for support of the girl and her baby, and her religious convictions.

If the girl decides to give the baby up for adoption, she must contend with some of the same issues as during the pregnancy, with the added feature of feelings of loss about her own baby. This may be a factor in depression, feelings of guilt, a later search for the infant, or other restitutive measures. In one institution, the young woman's task was aggravated by the punitiveness of the priest-director who made each girl care for her own baby in the adjacent nursery until she left three to five days postpartally, "to make her not have an out-of-wedlock baby again."

In order to keep the baby, the girl must have a supporting environment; its abscence often leads her into a move to another neighborhood or state, an impulsive marriage, or other unsatisfying arrangements. If she stays with her own parents, she may face continued regression and dependency, rejection, guilt, scapegoating, and perhaps the social taboos of the culture. A popular arrangement with the increased incidence of baby-keeping is for the girl to stay with her mother. This helps to magnify the conflict between them over her sexuality and dependency (Fisher, 1978; Sugar, 1979). The girl's arrested development may be reflected in her use of the infant as a transitional object, sleeping with the infant in her bed for years, or disallowing the grandparents to be involved with the infant in her presence (Sugar, 1979).

Early motherhood has been related very closely with the girl's inadequate education, economic deprivation, and, if married, with dissolution of her marriage. Of those who give birth at or before age 15, one third of the marriages ended in separation/divorce, in contrast to a ten percent dissolution rate in women who first became mothers after age 22. Marital instability is much greater among blacks than whites. Of those giving birth before age 16 who were ever married, nearly one third lived in poverty in 1967, which contrasted with one tenth in poverty in women who became mothers after age 22. For blacks, the probabilities of poverty related to age of marriage and motherhood were two to three times greater than those of whites in each age group. For women who gave birth before 16 years, nearly two thirds attained eight or fewer years of formal education, and only one fifth finished high school (Bacon, 1974).

Cutright (1973) felt that for blacks and whites the long-term economic effects of being pregnant premaritally were small. Coombs and Freedman (1970) found the opposite effect in white women who conceived before marriage: they remained disadvantaged economically for years.

PREJUDICE IN EDUCATION

At a critical time, when support is so vital, most schools reject the pregnant girl. In 1967, for the 17,000 school districts in the United States, there were 35 special school programs for the pregnant teenager; in 1972, the number was 225, and in 1975 there were 350 (Hansen et al, 1976).

Nationally, the schools that provide sex education supply facts on reproduction and venereal disease but don't dwell on the emotional or responsible aspects thereof (Castile, 1976; Calderone, 1966). Until recently, Louisiana law prohibited sex education in public schools, a distinction it shared for some years with no other state.

In 1976, Louisiana ranked second in the country in infant mortality, sixth in perinatal defects, seventh for illegitimate live births for girls under 20 (the total rate of 49 percent was made up of a 27 percent rate for whites and a 75 percent rate for nonwhites), second for syphilis in those under 14, and fourth for syphilis for those aged 15 to 19 (V.D. Fact Sheet, 1976; V.D. Statistical Letter, 1976). It is possible that deficient sex education contributed to these figures.

PREJUDICE IN INTERVENTION PROGRAMS

There have been a variety of programs designed for the pregnant adolescent, but few are comprehensive enough to involve primary and secondary prevention and later support for mother and infant for the desired minimum of three years postpartally.

When programs are short-term and short in funding, they got short-term results which are poor and militate against success and a sense of accomplishment. Sarrel (1967), LaBarre (1972), Osofsky et al (1973), Klerman and Jekel (1973), Furstenberg (1976), and Fisher (1978) among others have described some of these deficiencies and positive aspects with an indication of some drop in recidivism in some programs.

The programs must be comprehensive and start with the girl (who is vulnerable psychologically to risk-taking in conception); they must include abortion counselling, education about contraception, physiology (especially of reproduction) and nutrition, as well as general medical, dental, dietary, obstetric, and psychiatric services.

The girl at risk for conception may be quite different from the one at risk for early motherhood; separate specific profiles should be delineated for them as well as for the pregnancy repeater, the abortion repeater, and the repeat adolescent mother. Obviously, further research with improved research design is needed and should be built into the program.

SUCCESSFUL PROGRAMS

Perhaps the programs that do not continue or succeed have deficiencies in one of these areas due to prejudice or countertransference problems in the caregivers. The difficulties in offering continued suitable education and sex education to pregnant girls may be similarly based. Countertransference may be related among other things to their attitudes about the adolescent's sexuality, dependency, deviant behavior, ordinary developmental tasks of adolescence, the adults' ending reproductivity and/or their envy of, hostility to, or competition with, adolescents. An early reflection of this comes from the medical literature which gives the impression that a pregnancy in adolescence is a psychiatric disorder.

One of the earliest and most problematic areas is adequate funds for the sexually active teenager. This becomes involved in increasingly heated controversy the longer a program lasts, and especially so if the program calls for continuity until the infant of the young mother has progressed beyond the separation-individuation phase. At these junctures the community ire becomes most apparent to these girls.

An antiabortion ordinance in Buffalo, New York was barred from enforcement in November 1978. This would have required women seeking abortion to view photos of fetuses and be informed of all the possible consequences of an abortion—hemorrhage, sterility, psychological problems, and emotional disturbances. A similar ordinance was passed in Akron, Ohio (New York Times, 1978) while a parallel law in Louisiana is now being contested in court.

Another reflection of the countertransference problem is the statement that these girls get pregnant to receive ADC and to avoid working. A regularly occurring assumption indicating countertransference difficulty is the xenophobic remark that low income girls become pregnant because of indifference within their cultural patterns. This has been amply disqualified (Furstenberg, 1976). The absence of psychiatric and pediatric participation in framing PL94-142, and its exclusion of pregnant teenagers and adolescent mothers from consideration as handicapped youngsters for obtaining education or vocational skills, is another reflection of countertransference difficulty at a governmental level. This also implicates the legislative branch of the government for passivity and guilt in not having a national policy for children and adolescents. This is mirrored in the relative paucity of suitable schooling—sex education and education programs—especially for the pregnant and postpartal girl.

All adolescents are not similar; within the same age groups (of 12 to 14, 15 to 17, 18 to 21), there may be wide differences in development even if the adolescents are in the same developmental phase. Differences may occur in their psychosexual level, object relations, mourning of lost infantile objects (Sugar, 1969), identity, IQ, formal operations, academic achievement, work orientation, and/or ego and superego development, all of which will be influenced by family, culture, and SES.

Since many children are "surprise" children, even to married adults, it is strange to expect that adolescents should have any lesser percent of "surprises." The inability of the adolescent to plan ahead is often viewed as part of her psychopathology and this may well be the caregiver's and the psychiatrist's countertransference. Her difficulty in abstract ability may be specifically related to her growth (or its absence) in independence, separation-individuation, and sense of ownership of her body and genitals (see Chapter 3, this volume).

The above outlined foci for decision-making by the adolescent are not meant to be taken necessarily as signs of pathology if she has problems making these decisions. The usual teenager spends an inordinate amount of time agonizing over hair style or what clothes to wear; these kinds of decisions are often clearly involved in the development of separation from the mother. Considering such difficulties in making decisions, it should be apparent that in other matters in which the adolescent is less experienced, or which are more exciting, her decision-making would more likely by anxiety-ridden and incautious. Questions related to her sexuality or continence, contraception or pregnancy, delivery or abortion, and motherhood or adoption are highly cathected and are influenced by the presence or absence of psychopathology. They are also affected by the girl's intelligence level and her ability to abstract. We need to recall that half the population has an IQ of less than 100. Some with low IQs or those who are understimulated (especially the poor) may never achieve the ability for formal operations or abstract thinking (Piaget, 1972). Without the ability to plan ahead, decisions are most difficult. These items are frequently overlooked in the research design or program variables. Are these oversights and unrealistic expectations also countertransference-based?

The congressional legislation of 1978 providing for programs for pregnant adolescents and teenage mothers has yet to be implemented (see Chaper 12, this volume).

SUMMARY

This chapter has reviewed some of the facets of decision-making in adolescent motherhood. There are multiple determinants and differences in intelligence, nutritional state, socioeconomics, emotional development, culture, dynamics, and psychopathology involved in the decision to engage in coital activity, use contraception, become pregnant, abort, carry to term, give the baby up for adoption, or keep it.

Problems abound in the research of this arena, for example, separation of early from illegitimate motherhood, the lack of proper population comparisons, insufficient controls, the fact that population groups from different cultures and socioeconomic groups are insufficiently defined and separated, the fact that psychodynamics are confused with maturation or developmental arrests, and the knowledge that sociodynamic contributions are not entirely convincing and do not explain all.

Many problems have been short-lived and often focus only on facts of reproduction and contraception without providing counselling and comprehensive continued care.

Learning about causes and optimal solutions to problems is most difficult when observations and decisions are loaded with prejudices. Countertransference features interfere with understanding and awareness of the multiple tributaries to adolescent motherhood, research, and suitable intervention.

REFERENCES

Abernathy, V. and Abernathy, G. 1974. Risk for unwanted pregnancy among mentally ill adolescent girls. *Am. J. Orthopsychiatry* 44:442–450.

Alan Guttmacher Institute. 1976. *11 Million Teenagers.* New York: Planned Parenthood Federation of America.

Babikian, H. and Goldman, A. 1971. A study of teen-age pregnancy. *Am. J. Psychiatry* 128:755–760.

Bacon, L. 1974. Early motherhood, accelerated role transition, and social pathologies. *Soc. Forces* 52:333–341 (Spring).

Barglow, P., Bornstein, M., Exum, D., Wright, M. K. and Visotsky, H. M. 1968. Some psychiatric aspects of illegitimate pregnancy in early adolescence. *Am. J. Orthopsychiatry* 38:672–687.

Bonam, A. F. 1963. Psychoanalytic implications in treating unmarried mothers with narcissistic character structures. *Soc. Casework* 44:323–329.

Calderone, M. S. 1966. Sex and the adolescent. *Clin. Pediatr.* 5:171–174.

Castile, A. S. 1976. *School Health in America.* Kent, Ohio: American Health Association.

Coddington, R. D. 1979. Life Events Associated With Adolescent Pregnancies. *J. Clin. Psychiatry.* 40:180–185.

Coombs, L. C. and Freedman, R. 1970. Premarital pregnancy, child spacing and later economic achievement. *Popul. Stud.* 25:389–412.

Cutright, P. 1973. Timing the first birth: does it matter? *J. Marriage Fam.* 35:585–596.

Cutright, P. 1976. Family planning program effects on the fertility of low-income women. *Fam. Plann. Perspect.* 8:100–110.

Fisher, S. M. (1978. Teenage pregnancy: an anthropological, sociological and psychological overview. Presented at the American Academy of Child Psychiatry Meeting, October, 1978, San Diego, California.

Furstenberg, F. 1976. *Unplanned Parenthood.* New York: The Free Press, pp. 41, 42, 46, 49, 51, 56, 120.

Gabrielson, L. W., Gabrielson, I. W., Klerman, L. W., Currie, J. A., Tyler, N. C. and Jekel, S. F. 1970. Suicide attempts in a population pregnant as teenagers. *Am. J. Public Health* 60:2289–2301.

Gottschalk, L. A., Titchener, J. L., Piker, H. N. and Stewart, S. S. 1964. Psychosocial factors associated with pregnancy in adolescent girls: a preliminary report. *J. Nerv. Ment. Dis.* 138:524–534.

Hansen, C., Brown, M. and Trontell, M. 1976. Effects on adolescents of attending a special school. *J. Am. Diet. Assoc.* 68:538–541.

Johnson, C. L. 1974. Attitudes toward premarital sex and family planning for single-never pregnany teenage girls. *Adolescence* 9:255–259.

Kantner, J. F. and Zelnick, M. 1972. Sexual experiences of young unmarried women in the United States. *Fam. Plann. Perspect.* 4:9–18.

Kantner, J. F. and Zelnick, M. 1973. Contraception and pregnancy: experiences in young unmarried women in the United States. *Fam. Plann. Perspect.* 5:21–35.

Khlentzos, M. and Pagliaro, M. 1965. Observations from psychotherapy with unwed mothers. *Am. J. Orthopsychiatry* 35:779–786.

Kinch, R. A. H., Waring, M. P., Love, E. J. and McMahon, D. 1969. Some aspects of pediatric illegitimacy. *Am. J. Obstet. Gynecol.* 105:20–31.

Klerman, L. V. and Jekel, J. F. 1973. *School-Age Mother: Problems, Programs and Policy*. Hamden, Connecticut: Lennet Books.

LaBarre, M. 1972. Emotional crises of school-age girls during pregnancy and early motherhood. *J. Am. Acad. Child Psychiatry* 11:537-557.

Nadelson, C. 1974. Abortion counselling: focus on adolescent pregnancy. *Pediatrics* 54:765-769.

New York Times. 1978. December 17, Section I, p. 47.

Osofsky, H. J., Osofsky, J. D., Kendall, N. and Rajan, R. 1973. Adolescents as mothers: an interdisciplinary approach to a complex problem. *J. Youth Adol.* 2:233-249.

Pauker, J. 1971. Girls pregnant out of wedlock. *J. Operat. Psychiat.* 1:15-19.

Petersen, A. C. 1979. Female Pubertal Development. In M. Sugar (Ed.): *Female Adolescent Development*. New York: Brunner/Mazel.

Piaget, J. 1972. Intellectual evolution from adolescence to adulthood. *Hum. Devel.* 15:1-12.

Plionis, B. M. 1975. Adolescent pregnancy: review of the literature. *Soc. Work* 20:302-307.

Sarrel, P. M. 1967. The university hospital and the teenage unwed mother. *Am. J. Publ. Health* 57:1308-1313.

Sarrel, P. M. and Davis, C. A. 1966. The young unwed primipara, *Am. J. Obstet. Gynecol.* 95:722-725.

Schaffer, C. and Pine, F. 1972. Pregnancy, abortion, and the developmental tasks of adolescence. *J. Am. Acad. Child Psychiatry* 11:511-536.

Schlackman, V. 1966. Unmarried parenthood: an approach to social policy. *Soc. Casework* 47:494-501.

Sorensen, R. C. 1973. *Adolescent Sexuality in Contemporary America*. New York: World Press.

Sugar, M. 1979. Developmental Issues in Adolescent Motherhood. In M. Sugar (Ed.): *Female Adolescent Development*. New York: Brunner/Mazel.

U. S. News & World Report. 1978. June 26, pp. 59-60.

V. D. Fact Sheet. 1976. Ed. 33. U. S. Department of Health, Education, and Welfare Center for Disease Control. Washington, DC.

V. D. Statistical Letter #126. 1976. U. S. Department of Health, Education, and Welfare. Washington, D.C.

Vincent, C. E. 1961. *Unmarried Mothers*. New York: Free Press, p. 21.

Webb, G., Briggs, C. and Brown, R. 1972. A comprehensive adolescent maternity program in a community hospital. *Am. J. Obstet. Gynecol.* 113:511-523.

Williams, H. 1978. *The Times Picayune* (New Orleans). November 3, Section 3, p. 19.

Wynne, L. C. and Frader, L. 1979. Female Adolescence and the Family: A Historical View. In M. Sugar (Ed.): *Female Adolescent Development*. New York: Brunner/Mazel.

3

From (Re) Discovery to Ownership of the Vagina— A Contribution to the Explanation of Nonuse of Contraceptives in the Female Adolescent

MOISY SHOPPER

The nonuse of contraceptives in sexually active adolescent girls is a problem of major social, economic, and psychological magnitude with adverse ramifications that can continue into succeeding generations. This chapter focuses on the significant intrapsychic and developmental factors which might aid in understanding the phenomena of nonuse. In brief, a developmental sequence in adolescent female sexuality is postulated: the (re)discovery (Shopper, 1979) to ownership of the genitalia which militates *against* the use of contraceptives during early sexual activity. Understanding the nature of this developmental sequence could lead to practices which would increase contraceptive use before and/or concomitant with initial adolescent sexual activity.

In their 1971 survey, Shah and associates (1975) asked females aged 15 to 19 their reasons for not using contraception. The answers: "wrong time of the month" (39.7 percent), "low risk of pregnancy" (30.9 percent), "contraceptives unavailable" (30.5 percent), "interferes with pleasure" (23.7 percent), "moral or medical objection" (12.5 percent), "didn't mind getting pregnant" (9.3 percent), and "wanted a baby" (6.5 percent). Unfortunately, no attempt was made to ascertain which are mere rationalizations and which are serious reasons. If the answers are rationalizations, one must look for other motivations (conscious or unconscious) and direct the preventive programs toward the true causes for nonuse. On the other hand, if these are accepted as nonrationalized true reasons, perhaps effective prevention of adolescent pregnancy might include better education and more adequate service programs.

Indeed, the Alan Guttmacher Institute (1976) takes this exact approach. In their view, improvements would follow by offering better sex education to teenagers. This would include birth control and contraception, accessibility of birth control services for teenagers within easy traveling of the teenager's residence, increased federal funding for research in reproductive and contraceptive planning, and knowledge of available abortion services. One can hardly fault Planned Parenthood for embarking on a program in which they have both expertise and success, namely, educational planning and delivery of services. However, it is of interest and significance that the development of the female adolescent is nowhere considered from a psychological standpoint, but merely from an epidemiologic and physiologic standpoint. To the extent that mental processes are considered, they are mainly of a cognitive nature. While cognition is not to be downplayed, to make it the entire story is an error. Clinical experience provides daily instances where there is full cognitive awareness and available opportunities for contraception, but teenage pregnancies ensue nevertheless.

The major factor in adolescent contraceptive nonuse discussed by Nadelson and associates (1978) is the conscious and/or unconscious motivation to become pregnant. They outlined some of the character and personal qualities needed for the use of contraceptives and said, "Since the use of contraception implies acknowledgment of, and responsibility for, sexuality, it may not be consistent with the ego development of adolescence." In their pilot study of adolescent sexuality, they noted that adolescents who had courses on sexual information and education were not able to integrate and utilize this knowledge, nor did it build toward the use of contraceptives.

This chapter focuses on those special intermediary developmental tasks of female adolescence which need to be traversed successfully in order for the teenager to effectively and consistently use the "better sex education" and "available services." This chapter proposes to (1) define the psychological concept of ownership and demonstrate its utility, (2) to clarify the role of "ownership of the genital" as an intermediary phase in female sexual development, (3) to show the usefulness of the concept of "psychological ownership of the genital" in elucidating the problem of contraceptive nonuse among sexually active teenagers, and (4) to offer some tentative suggestsions which may increase contraceptive use and decrease the time lag between initiation of sexual activity and initiation of contraceptive use.

CONCEPT OF OWNERSHIP AND ITS DEVELOPMENTAL LINE

The term *ownership* is being used in a psychological context to denote not only possession but an exclusive possession and control that allows the child almost full choice as to what and how to manage this possession (Winnicott, 1953). The concept of possession has its developmental roots in the differentiation of the self from the mother-child symbiosis and the differentiation of the "me" from the "not me", that is, the inanimate environment. Something "not of me" becomes "mine" because I have declared it to be so and have given it a "mine" designation. Hopefully this will be accepted rather than challenged by the child's outside world. While the consensual validation of "mine" is desirable, it is not essential to the concept of "mine."

Bergman (1980) noted that "Around the rapprochement crisis we found an interesting cluster of phenomena: (1) increased independent functioning; (2) greater self-assertiveness; (3) increased use of the word "mine"; (4) increased availability and wish to play at some distance from mother; (5) increased awareness of bodily sensations . . . and (6) competitiveness over possession being the most frequent source of anger." She observed that there is "an increased need to defend one's possessions [concomitant] with one's growing awareness of self." This is frequently manifested by the child crying out "mine!" in a mixture of rage, determination, panic, and assertiveness.

During the second year of life, battles over the "not me but mine" possession are found in the toddler's and parents' attitudes toward clothes. Clothes are experienced as part of the self. Hats, shoes, jewelry, ties, and other easy-off/easy-on clothes are play materials for the child's eager experimentation in "putting themselves in someone else's shoes", that is, being another self. One's own clothes seem to hold all the aspects of one's own self, one's body, one's integrity and identity (Bergman, 1980).

As the toddler achieves a growing sense of separateness and individuation from the mother, the mother begins to demand that the child's autonomous functioning, particularly in the excretory sphere, be brought under the control of the child and then of the parent. This is accomplished in stages. First the mother "trains" the child to bring its autonomous physiologic functioning under its own autonomous conscious and deliberate control. The second step is to bring this function under the mother's control in terms of her timing, place, and method. The final stage is the incorporation of the parental control into one's self—the maturing from a sphincter morality to an internalized identification with the parent.

This struggle to bring the child's egocentric/autonomous functioning more and more under parental control continues throughout the course of the child's development. In latency, for example, it concerns the ownership of the child's body, namely, whether or not to take a bath, how long to stay in the bath, whether to wash hands and face, or brush, cut, and style hair. Concerning oral matters, although the child is autonomous, it is nevertheless taught how much it is allowed to put into its mouth at any one time politely, whether to talk when chewing, how fast to eat, and other accoutrements of proper manners for that household.

Often, during the second separation and individuation phase in adolescence, to the consternation and opposition of the parents, the adolescent claims ownership of the body and its functioning, and progresses to make her own decisions regarding bodily hygiene, clothing style, sleeping and eating patterns, etc. It is as though the adolescent were saying that she not only can control her body, but she is the *one and only person* who will decide how, when, and where to control that body, a function previously requisitioned by the parents during earlier development.

A common clinical example is the mother-daughter interaction concerning the daughter's hair. Initially, it is the mother who decides everything about the girl's hair style, length, curl, and appearance. A scene of idyllic mother-daughter harmony is the mother tenderly and lovingly brushing her daughter's hair, with the latter's full approval and pleasure. With the approach of adolescence, the girl begins to voice her own wishes regarding her hair style, frequently influenced by her mother. As Rosenbaum (1979) pointed out, "hair tends to be one of the ongoing battlegrounds where the conflict of control, as well as separation-individuation, is fought between mothers and daughters. During adolescence, a girl tends to move into *autonomous ownership of this body part*" (italics mine). This takeover of ownership of her body occurs in a piecemeal fashion with similar struggles over control focusing on fingernails and nail polish, eyes and eye make-up, ears and ear-piercing, going bra-less, total body weight, bathing suits, jeans, etc.

In the past there were specific issues which almost qualified as a symbolic rite of passage: for example, when a girl could wear high-heeled shoes. More recently, the focus was on ear-piercing, smoking in the house, going bra-less, and alcohol use. Many of the seemingly outlandish things the adolescent wears or does are not just to be rebellious and negative to the parental authority, but to declare and define for herself the extent of her bodily ownership. It is as though she feels she must wrest control of her body from the parents, and flagrantly assert that she and only she controls and owns her body. As with many issues in adolescence, these can become an intense source of parent/child conflict or they may proceed relatively conflict-free.

A vestigial rite of passage present currently is the father escorting his daughter down the aisle, "giving the bride away" to his future son-in-law. In this symbolic act, the father relinquishes his "ownership" of his daughter, and her virginity passes from his protection to that of the husband who will similarly protect her virtue and good name.

Laufer (1968), in his classic study, reported several adolescents whose pathologic conflicts concerning masturbation were such as to lead them to regard their bodies as alien and foreign: ". . . a central feature is the extent to which they dissociated their minds from their bodies and from the sensations arising in their bodies. They (both male and female adolescents) felt that they must not have feelings and viewed the internalized mother as the person who was responsible for the control of their feelings. . . . Both felt as though their mothers were giving them permission to experience feelings; but they also felt that she could withdraw this permission at any time, and their body and its sensations had to be *disowned*" (italics mine). As a result of their conflicts, they could not acknowledge, accept, experience, or *own* their genitals and their accompanying sensations and masturbatory urges. Laufer (1968) spoke of this situation as "an intrapsychic deadlock" of the adolescent process.

TOILET TRAINING, MENSTRUATION, AND VAGINAL OWNERSHIP

In the course of the toilet training of the girl, there is a tendency for mothers to train her as though the excretory-genital area was an undifferentiated one, that is, offering her a cloacal theory (Shopper, 1967). Frequently, the term "vagina" is given to the girl as a generic term for the area between her legs and refers in an undifferentiated fashion to the combined genital and excretory organs. As pointed out by Kleeman (1975) "vagina" may be used by parent and/or child to refer to the conglomerate of vulva, labia, clitoris, urethral meatus, vagina, and rectum. Vaginal sensations and vaginal stimulation, to the extent that they are present, are not clearly localized to the vagina but are diffuse and subsumed under its anatomic and physiologic neighbors, bladder and rectum. Later, in adolescence, the onset of menstruation allows the vagina to receive some specific awareness and thus aids in the differentiation process for the female (Shopper, 1967). Kestenberg (1961) has pointed to menarche as being "an organizing experience" for the female adolescent. Organization and differentiation proceed together as the young girl crystalizes the differentiation of (1) the urinary opening, its contents and its function from (2) the vaginal function, its contents and its opening from (3) the rectal functioning, its content and its opening.

However, as I pointed out earlier (Shopper, 1979), differentiation certainly aids but does not guarantee the "(re)discovery" of the vagina. The mother and/or other women provide the pubescent girl with menstrual information, since menstruation requires acknowledgment and information, particularly as it is a function beyond the girl's control. At best, she can keep a dated record of her menses, their length, and what bodily sensations (cramps, bloating, etc.) precede or occur during the flow. While menstruation focuses on the vagina and helps distinguish the vagina and the vaginal opening from its anatomic and physiologic neighbors, during the menstrual flow the vagina functions as a relatively passive and sensationless organ. To a large extent, menstruation duplicates for the girl all of the aspects of her earlier toilet training with her mother. As in the past, the menstruating girl simply brings her menses and her vagina under the control and ownership of the mother, just as she did earlier with her bladder and rectum.

Clinically, it is the mother who is usually the first to be told of the onset of menses. The initial maternal advice regarding use/nonuse of tampons, napkins, baths, etc., are usually obeyed by the young girl for quite some time. In addition to this compliance, the mother may often keep track of her daughter's periods, exchange menstrual experiences (for example, pain or discomfort) and share a common supply of napkins. Thus, as with the earlier issue of toileting, her vaginal functions, such as menses, are brought under the control and ownership of the mother.

This may be further enhanced through the gynecologic experience. In case of vaginal or menstrual dysfunction (such as discharge), when a visit to the gynecologist is indicated, it is the rare mother and rare daughter that would not utilize the same gynecologist, namely the mother's.

It is only when the girl takes active control over her vagina that the girl progresses to the vagina as "part of self that is owned by me," that is, "mine." When tampons have been deliberately overlooked by the mother in her menstrual hygiene instructions or when tampons have been specifically or tacitly condemned, the use of vaginal tampons by the daughter is a developmental step toward the ownership of her vagina and making her vagina more of a "mine" possession. Although it is an important developmental step, it is however a limited one, pertaining *only* to the time of menstrual flow and only to the vagina as a passive excretory passage (for the shedded decidua) rather than to the vagina as an *active* sexual organ with exciting sensations, vaginal lubrication, and the capacity for intercourse and orgastic discharge. What is being postulated is an intermediary stage of *passive vaginal ownership* which follows vaginal (re)discovery but precedes active vaginal ownership. The criteria for vaginal "passivity" is that (1) it functions as a passive conduit in the passive excretory process of the menstrual flow, (2) it functions passively in a physiologic sense, and (3) it is passive with respect to sensations originating in the vagina. It is when the adolescent girl departs from mother's control and teachings, via changed menstrual hygiene techniques,[1] that she assumes ownership of her vagina, albeit a passive vagina.

[1] These changes may take the form of previously prohibited or scorned tampons, douches, deodorants, etc.

In their discussions of menstrual hygiene, some mothers do inform their daughters of tampons, indicate their approval, and extol their convenience. Despite this "Good Housekeeping Seal of Approval" from mother, the girl may regard the tampon as "yucky" and refuse to use one for several years (Clark, personal communication, 1980). I would hypothesize that the teenager intuitively knew that she was not ready emotionally to accept even "passive ownership" of this area of her body. This would represent the psychosexual moratorium of adolescence (Shopper, 1979) initiated and protected by the adolescent. It is as though the teenager intuitively recognizes that the (re)discovery of her vagina and taking claim to its ownership is something for which she currently lacks the emotional capacity to manage and had best postpone.

REGRESSIVE LOSS OF OWNERSHIP OF ONE'S BODY

In some instances, adequate adaptation to a situation involves the capacity to tolerate and even to value the loss of bodily ownership, no matter how hard won or painstakingly attained. The exigencies of medical examination, procedures, and surgery demand a relinquishment of control *and* ownership over one's body. For a while the body "belongs" to the x-ray technician, the nurse, the surgeon, the endoscopist, etc. It is the regressive nonownership of one's own body that makes being a patient so difficult for some, and so gratifying to others. To attain high degrees of proficiency in certain sports, in dance, or in musical performance, one must, in the course of being taught, learn to do it the teacher's way. In effect, it means to let the teacher control and own the apprentice's body and, through repetition and practice, produce an automatized internalization of this ownership. For the purpose of heightened performance, agreement to temporary and controlled regression to a state of nonownership of one's body and the externalization of body ownership is readily seen in symphony orchestras, choruses, the cast of a play, the members of a sports team, and, most glaringly, in the basic training procedures of the armed services. Again, for some the loss of body ownership is discomforting while for others it is a source of gratification.

VAGINAL OWNERSHIP AND THE BOYFRIEND

In the developmental line to ownership of her vagina, the virginal girl is hampered by the difficulty of localizing diffuse and indefinite sensations. When Rosenbaum (1979) asked nonpatient adolescent girls about their sexual excitement (being "horny"), "Only the girls who had had genital sexual experiences would even mention genital sensations, usually upon direct questioning stating,

'It's a lustful feeling. I guess most girls don't feel much and are not aware of any feelings down there.' " It is as though the participation of the male is necessary to stimulate a focused awareness of sexual arousal and excitement. However, this may have a significant defensive function for the girl in that her sexual arousal becomes a shared responsibility with the boyfriend. In many cases he is perceived as more responsible than she, simply because he may have taken the initiative, been somewhat more knowledgeable and forceful, and his actions conformed to the cultural stereotype of the sex-crazed male seducing/raping the innocent, unwilling female. In any case, the participation of the boyfriend facilitates a disavowal of her responsibility and participation in her sexual arousal, and increases her tendency to feel that she is consciously or unconsciously the victim of her boyfriend's passions. In addition, participation by the boyfriend carries connotations of social approval in that heterosexual sex is an acceptable "grown-up" activity, as compared with the view of masturbation as more childish, immature, and asocial.

CLINICAL ILLUSTRATION

The patient described her recent visit to the gynecologist to be fitted for a diaphragm. Once before she had one, but discarded it. This time she went because her current boyfriend dislikes condoms and she felt that foam would be too messy and not to her liking.

Unlike the previous time, she felt that she had the courage to ask the gynecologist if the diaphragm would remain in place even when she moved. He assured her it would. However, she felt he did not understand her question because what she was referring to was not to movement in the sense of physical movement, like walking or running but internal movement, that is, by her pelvic and vaginal muscles. The gynecologist jokingly said that at last he had found a Jewish woman who moves. She was very pleased at this compliment and felt reassured that the diaphragm would not be dislodged during "movement." She was concerned about a correct fit because on return for a checkup with the diaphragm in place (after her first diaphragm experience) she saw the associate of the original doctor who told her the diaphragm was too small and she needed a larger size. She never questioned him or returned for a clarification of the disagreement between the two doctors. Presently, to be absolutely certain, she asked the doctor to try the larger size, which he did, and found himself in agreement with his own earlier opinion.

She felt very pleased with the diaphragm and felt it was something she could share with her boyfriend in the sense of inserting it in his presence, and perhaps at sometime in the future asking him to insert it for her. In this way they would be "sharing the responsibility" for the contraception.

This is an example of a woman who is now comfortable with her sense of ownership of her genitals and whose ownership extends to taking responsibility for its sexual excitement and activation. In her earlier encounters with the gynecologist and his associate, she was too ill at ease to fully resolve the question regarding her proper diaphragm size, much less ask additional questions. In this instance she did not hesitate to openly confront this issue, as well as openly acknowledge her sexuality to the gynecologist.

Although she takes responsibility for her sexual arousal and responsibility for the ownership of her genitals, she also wishes to share the responsibility for contraception and so looks forward to her boyfriend partaking in the insertion process. While it is her diaphragm, her cervix, and her vagina, he nevertheless can participate to this extent. She was also very pleased that he offered to pay the fee for her visit to the gynecologist. This sharing of responsibility *with* the boyfriend is far different from an abdication of responsibility *to* the boyfriend, which would be a sharing in name more than in actuality.

MASTURBATION

In the developmental line to ownership of one's vagina *and its associated sexuality*, there are two possible routes: one proceeding through self-masturbation, the other proceeding through boyfriend-masturbation and/or boyfriend intercourse. Self-masturbation as the transition step has several advantages in that sexual stimulation, being self-initiated and self-induced, does not offer many escapes from assuming responsibility for such arousal and orgasm.[2] It also serves to familiarize the girl with her own genitalia, her capacity for excitement, and her degree of control of such excitement. Masturbation also offers her the benefits of readily available sexual discharge without the problems and consequences of heterosexual intercourse: pregnancy, venereal disease, a "bad reputation," discovery as well as the vicissitudes of complicated boyfriend/girlfriend problems.

In examining three groups of teenagers in Oakland, Goldsmith and associates (1972) found that (1) the contraceptor group (that is, those new patients never pregnant attending a Planned Parenthood Teen Clinic) were least anxious about masturbation compared with (2) a group seeking abortion for a problem pregnancy and (3) the group who carried a pregnancy to term. The authors

---

[2] It is true that the many forms of unconscious masturbatory activities and masturbatory equivalents do offer just such an escape in that neither the self-initiation, the activity, nor the pleasure is consciously perceived and/or acknowledged. What I am speaking of here is the conscious and deliberately initiated genital masturbatory activity.

concluded that this was one of many indications of the contraceptors' greater acceptance of their sexuality. However, they noted that for all groups, masturbation was viewed "with more censure than intercourse, reflecting a strong social taboo against the common practice and alternate sexual outlet."

Clower (1975) specifically stated, "The adolescent girl needs to masturbate enough to reinforce the awareness of her genitality, especially to experience vaginal lubrication and excitement spreading from the clitoris. She must not masturbate so much that her sexual gratification is fixed on her own body and fantasies of being able to satisfy herself are promoted at the expense of accepting the need for vaginal penetration and coitus."

It would seem that masturbation, while itself fraught with certain anxieties and dangers, is far to be preferred to sexual intercourse as the developmental route to ownership of the genital. Though concerned, lest the girl find masturbation so satisfying and so narcissistically fixating as to preclude or divert the girl from sexual intercourse, Clower may be overstating her case. Masturbation need not necessarily divert the girl from object relationships nor from heterosexuality, but may allow her a less complicated, less dangerous outlet for sexual discharge (for which she is physiologically ready) and avoidance of the more complicated aspects of intercourse and object relatedness for which she may not have sufficient maturity. Having taken an active role in initiating her own masturbation and mastering its frequency, fantasies, and course, she is better able to cope with her boyfriend and his pressures toward sexual intercourse. She has considerably less need to defensively regress to a state of nonownership of her body and genitals in order to avoid acknowledging her participation in intercourse and sexuality. The girl who accepts her need to masturbate, her genitals, and her sexuality has a less defensive need to transfer ownership of her genitals to her boyfriend. With such a transfer comes a reliance on the boyfriend for contraceptive precautions (if they are not already totally denied) with a concomitant abdication of her own responsibility for contraception.

In some instances it is just such masturbatory inhibitions that preclude the use of intravaginal contraceptives. It is as though the girl cannot take any responsibility for inserting something into her vagina "that doesn't belong there," such as a diaphragm or foam. If the boyfriend inserts his penis she can reason "it belongs there" in the sense that heterosexuality is good and intercourse is a mature, adult activity. But if the adolescent girl reasons "it doesn't belong there," she didn't put it there, and besides "it's his fault/doing." For these girls the pill is preferable since it totally avoids these vaginal issues.

Borowitz (1973), while discussing the adolescent male only, pointed out the developmental achievement represented by the capacity to masturbate alone. It "provides a setting in which working through by the use of fantasies of preadolescent self and object representations and modes of drive discharge may occur." However, he did not discuss the concept of ownership of the genital, which may not be as significant or clearly definable a factor in the boy as in the adolescent girl.

EDUCATION

Better sex education as advocated by Planned Parenthood cannot only be improved by the inclusion of birth control information, but can be made "better" by discussion of "those topics least often (discussed) both at school and at home—orgasm and masturbation" (Goldsmith et al, 1972). This high degree of avoidance of the sexual-pleasurable in contrast to the sexual-reproductive is to be found even in anatomic and physiologic discussions. For example, the girl's genital is labeled "the vagina" as though it subsumes the labia and the clitoris, and thus no further mention need be made of their presence nor of their nonreproductive, nonmenstrual function. Labia and clitoris function exclusively in the sexual-pleasurable realm. To acknowledge them anatomically is to acknowledge the pleasurable capacity inherent in sexual activity and inherent in the girl's anatomy. Unlike the vagina, which has multiple functions (obstetric, menstrual, reproductive, and pleasurable/orgastic), the clitoris and labia are clearly differentiated from the vagina proper and have a unitary function—pleasurable/orgastic. Thus, discussions of the vagina may be extensive and intensive and still avoid the pleasurable/orgastic, such cannot be the case with the labia and clitoris.

The point of all this is to emphasize that anatomic and physiologic discussions should include those organs and functions of the pleasurable/orgastic realm. This acknowledges that the genitals are menstrual organs which require both knowledge of their function and certain care, and simultaneously acknowledges that the genitals are pleasure/orgasm organs which also require specific knowledge of their function and care. The use/nonuse, control of excitation-arousal, masturbation and/or intercourse, and appropriate birth control measures are all issues related to the pleasure/orgasm realm and therefore are worthy and necessary topics for sexual education curriculum.

In addition to better naming of anatomic parts (Lerner, 1976) and the implications thereof, the combined effects of personal repression, cultural suppression, and perceptual invisibility need to be overcome, both cognitively and educationally. Many texts that discuss sexual or menstrual matters use schematic diagrams of the genitals. Although diagrams are clear and useful as teaching devices, and although they focus on the significant details, the absence of photographs and/or realistic sketches supports the maintenance of secrecy, mystery, and ignorance. Similarly, the use of teaching manikins would be an educational advantage, providing three-dimensional clarity. The genital manikin, in a sense dehumanized and not being a part of a greater human anatomy model, offers a transient defense against sexual arousal and other affects (negative or positive) when cognitive information is acquired.

Furthermore, advocacy of the girl's use of a hand-held mirror to better view her own genitals is necessary.[3] The actual viewing of her own genitals provides for the adolescent girl something readily achieved by the average boy many years earlier—a sense of firm sexual identity (Greenacre, 1958). It is difficult for the girl to know about her own genitals and take responsibility for their use (as in contraception) if she has never seen them, or if, daring to look, the looking and the knowledge so gained are fraught with shame and a sense of wrongdoing. Not seeing her own genitals, and frequently too inhibited to manually explore herself, the girl must await the genital petting activities of her boyfriend to be provided with direct tactile knowledge of her genitals. However educational this is, its cognitive value is often lost in the flood of sexual affects and excitement. Combined visual-tactile self-examination as an approved educational exercise would be relatively free of the flooding sexual excitement and would provide two perceptual modalities for the acquisition of knowledge.

Tradition has it that only the gynecologist has the right to touch and view the female genitalia, except on the delivery table when, at the woman's request, a mirror can be positioned so that she can watch herself deliver her child. What I am suggesting is that physicians, nurses, sex educators, and parents advocate as an educational practice the girl's use of a mirror to inspect her genitals. This would facilitate the incorporation of her genitalia into her body image and her sexual identity, and would facilitate the ownership of her genitalia as an integrated part of her total body and self. By whom and where such curriculum is to be taught—home, school, church, agency, parents, physicians, or educators—is a topic too large and complicated for this chapter.

However, many in the Women's Movement have long advocated "self-help," "taking back our bodies," and similar concepts, which are presented more from a political than a psychological stance. Nevertheless, they have advocated the use of a hand-held mirror for self knowledge as well as the self-use of a speculum so that the vaginal canal and cervix could be viewed (Rennie and Grimstead, 1975). In the context of pathology, many young women exposed to diethylsilbesterol (DES) reported being helped by being shown slides of normal vaginal mucosa and the DES-induced pathologic adenosis. It demystified the pathologic features and provided an opportunity for a greater degree of intellectual mastery of an anxious and frightening situation.

---

[3] In many ways it doesn't make educational sense that adolescent women should be shielded from photographs of their own genitalia presented in an educational context, when magazines such as *Penthouse* and *Playboy* present photographs not only of the woman's genitals but of the sexually seductively-posed woman.

THE ISSUE OF DENIAL

Many authors have noted the prevalent use of denial mechanisms in sexually active teenagers regarding the possibility of a subsequent unwanted pregnancy. While they have the cognitive information needed to conclude that unprotected intercourse will result eventually in a pregnancy and are able even to apply that knowledge to their peers' activities, they nevertheless maintain in thought, deed, and fantasy that they *personally* will not become pregnant. Such massive denial about so significant a matter might be ascribed to the transient regressive breaks in reality testing typical of adolescent development. Some would explain that the strength and pressure of sexual urges cause regression in logical thinking, allowing wishful thinking to supplant reason and reality. Or, similarly, the pressure for immediate gratification overwhelms consideration of long-term consequences. What is certain is that the need to believe that they personally won't become pregnant readily leads to the failure to acquire adequate and accurate knowledge. It also leads to the creation and/or perpetuation of factual misconceptions and inaccurate fantasies, such as one "can't get pregnant in certain positions," or one "can't get pregnant if sex is only occasional," among others.

This viewpoint assumes that the denial mechanism is primary and thus "causes" the resulting factual inaccuracies, which in turn precludes effective contraception. I propose that the inability to use effective contraception is not the result of denial mechanisms, but is, rather, primary and etiologic. The urge to be sexually active, an urge based both on biological id factors *and* developmental progressions, comes into conflict with the need to avoid pregnancy and to use contraception. When the conflict is decided in favor of the former, as it frequently is, denial mechanisms are needed to support the former and to devaluate and dismiss the latter. Thus, I see the denial mechanisms not as a causative factor, but, as with all defense mechanisms, a relief from the painfulness and anxiety of the conflict by invalidation of the weight of reality and long-term considerations.

To our understanding of the motivations for using denial, another should be added: the average adolescent girl does not own her genital, and therefore does not feel the need (1) to be responsible for how it is used; (2) have accurate and informed knowledge concerning its use; (3) or know the consequences of such use. To obtain contraception, whether from physician, birth control clinic, or drug store counter, necessitates acknowledgement and acceptance of her sexuality and her genitals, and thus runs counter to the use of denial mechanisms or, to be more accurate, makes denial mechanisms unnecessary. Her denial is not simply ignorance and misunderstanding combined with the regressive vicissitudes of the adolescent process, but is a concomitant of an intermediary developmental step *prior* to the attainment of her sense of genital ownership.

CLINICAL ILLUSTRATION

A college student entered treatment complaining of depression, which she recognized was precipitated by leaving her home and mother. During the initial interview she referred to her mother as being the director of a hospital, unaware that this was a slip (I was unaware that this was inaccurate). In actuality her mother was a director of a small department of a nonmedical nature. Reputedly, she was the most powerful administrative figure in the hospital, which the patient ascribed to a combination of nerve, wit, ambition, and seniority. As a child, the patient was given ballet, speech, and piano lessons and was taught to be a compliant and efficient cook and housekeeper. The mother was quite controlling and had the patient's nose "fixed" as well as her ears pinned back (even though the patient's long hair style did not leave the ears exposed).

The patient realized that her boyfriend similarly exploited and mistreated her but she needed him for security, closeness, and love. She quickly became pregnant (she left birth control to him) and quickly had an abortion. This reactivated her recall of the mother-initiated surgery where her body was judged to be faulty/unacceptable and the surgeon "would make it all better." The degree to which she felt herself and her body still controlled by her mother became increasingly apparent and amazing to her. However, in this current instance she was the one who judged the pregnancy unacceptable, and *she* decided on the abortion and made all the arrangements. Her parents had no knowledge of the abortion and she was insistent that her boyfriel not know of or participate supportively in the abortion, all in an attempt to claim ownership to her own body.

The therapeutic efforts to help her take claim to her own body, to her own self, and to her own future professional plans occupied a major portion of her treatment. Nevertheless, despite her excellent cognitive knowledge of conception, birth control, *and* abortion, there were additional episodes of unprotected sexual intercourse where she claimed drunkness as an excuse—"I didn't know what I was doing"—even though she had resolved to no longer have anything to do with the exploitative, impregnating exboyfriend.

In addition to other dynamic factors, I wish to emphasize that during these inebriated states, she once more ceded to the boyfriend the control of her body and genitals, the boyfriend representing the maternal imago. Her sense of genital ownership increased as the sadomasochistic, controlling, intrusive relationship with the mother was loosened and relinquished.

THE GYNECOLOGIST AND FIRST OFFICE VISIT

From my clinical experience and conversation with friends and colleagues who are the parents of daughters, it seems that the first visit to the gynecologist usually occurs as a result of some pathology—vaginal discharge, menstrual disturbances, or abnormalities in development. These visits are handled on the already existing model of pediatric office visits, namely, the child informs the parent of the disturbance, and the parent decides whether it requires pediatric care and the nature of the care needed (a telephone call or visit). The mother calls for the appointment and accompanies her child to the pediatrician. The mother may or may not give the history of the presenting complaint and may or may not be present during the examination of the child, but is the person to whom the pediatrician speaks concerning the findings, diagnosis, and treatment recommendations. This paradigm will vary depending on the mother's and pediatrician's need and/or wish to see the child patient as an autonomous, intelligent, and separate individual as opposed to someone with an undifferentiated or appendage status.

With the development of adolescent medicine as a subspecialty within pediatrics, there is a growing tendency to treat the adolescent more and more on the paradigm of an adult patient vis-à-vis an internist, that is, with parental knowledge and participation being a variable option for both the adolescent and the physician. Similarly, the gynecologist, and the extent that he or she is aware of the psychological developmental issues of adolescence, will follow either the pediatric model or the adult-internist model, or an idiosyncratic blend of each paradigm.

In some instances, the pediatric paradigm is to be preferred by all parties since it facilitates the diagnosis and treatment of the condition, and alleviates the teenager's anxiety through the use of a familiar and expected procedure. The pediatric model is particularly appropriate and useful when the teenager is at the developmental level where the genitals are dormant[4] and are owned by the mother. Her presence during history taking and at the pelvic examination would relieve the teenager's apprehension, not only to minimize the heterosexual seductive aspects (as with a male gynecologist), but also because the mother as owner of her daughter's genitals would ensure that no harm would befall her during the examination; and that any excitement/arousal would be immediately controlled and extinguished. Similarly, the teenager would appreciate her mother's involvement/interest in the treatment and recommendations, particularly because any genital touching, manipulations, and insertions must meet with maternal approval. It is the current mother's current approval to touch that must counteract the mother-of-the-past's disapproval and prohibitions of touching.

In the absence of specific genital pathology, most adolescents do not seek out a gynecologist simply because they have beome young women. Rather, their first visit is postponed until there is a need basis—sexual information and/or

---

[4] Dormancy refers here to sexual genital dormancy. Although menstruation may have been established as a regular occurrence, it is conceived as a passive excretory activity, that is, not of the sexual-pleasure realm.

birth control.[5] More often than not, the adult-internist model is utilized. The adolescent evaluates and decides whether to go, makes an appointment, goes unaccompanied (or with peer or mother surrogate), gives the history in privacy, is examined with typical regard for privacy and modesty accorded an adult, is informed of the findings, diagnosis, and treatment recommendations, is given the oppotunity to ask questions, and *her wishes for privacy and confidentiality are respected*.

To proceed in this more adult paradigm requires a degree of maturity most often absent in the teenager just initiating her sexual activity. The adult paradigm I believe is based on the adolescent's growing sense of individuation, her wish to assume greater control and care of her body, and her progress in separating emotionally from her mother. Frequently, a geographic move to an out-of-town school, summer camp, etc. seems to represent in a concrete way an escape or the attainment of freedom from the mother's control and sphere of influence. It is as though the girl, living under her mother's roof and within her house, feels that she herself is part and parcel of all that mother owns and controls.[6] Under these circumstances, there would be a greater tendency for the girl to utilize the pediatric model.

The major disadvantage of the pediatric model for the developing adolescent is that it does not provide for privacy and confidentiality. If a teenager makes a request of the mother to see the gynecologist and does not reveal to the mother the nature of the complaint, the average mother will assume (1) the teenager is dreadfully ill ("unlikely"); (2) the teenager is pregnant or thinks she might be ("a distinct albeit dreadful possibility"); or (3) the teenager is sexually active and wants contraception ("I appreciate the forethought but she's too young"). All these responses will frequently exacerbate mother/daughter conflicts.

The teenager who wants to see a gynecologist to secure contraception and/or information faces difficult options. If she has to follow the pediatric model and report to the mother, but wishes to keep private the birth control purpose of her visit, she has to lie and manufacture a hint of genital pathology (for example, vaginal discharge) to use as a cover story and allay her mother's apprehension, curiosity, and fantasies about her sexual activity. Or she could call her mother's gynecologist and request an appointment without her mother's knowledge. Here she runs the risk of breaches of confidentiality: if any of her

---

[5] I omit from the discussion those adolescents whose first visit is for a pregnancy or pregnancy testing, since my emphasis is on developmental vicissitudes as they pertain to the *prevention* of pregnancy.

[6] The girl often wonders where she could hide her pills, diaphragm, etc. with the certainty that her mother wouldn't find it. It is as though, at this stage of her development, she cannot envision any nook or cranny of her body or room safe enough from mother's intrusive and watchful eye, that is, that does not belong to mother.

mother's friends would see her unaccompanied at the gynecologist's office, if the parents be billed for the visit even though she requested to pay for it herself, if the nurses, receptionist, or gynecologist would inadvertently refer to her visit during the mother's next visit. Even if all in the office were reasonably sensitive to the daughter's need for confidentiality, the daughter would still be apprehensive about a slip-up simply because she and her mother shared the same gynecologist.[7] It may also be that in actuality and/or in fantasy the gynecologist is caught in a conflict of interest because his or her initial and primary doctor/patient relationship is with the mother, and in identification with her parenting role (Shopper, 1979) may wish to postpone and/or condemn precocious sexual intercourse. It should be understood that in the daughter's mind the mother's gynecologist would (1) represent the parental viewpoint (that is, condemning), (2) be clearly identified with the mother's viewpoint, and (3) be loyal to the mother. Rather than enhancing the daughter's separation from the mother and affirming her sexual maturation and feminine identity, the gynecologic visit may continue the past, if the gynecologist is the mother's. For the adult-internist model to prevail, the gynecologist has to be one who is *not* the mother's *nor* the mother's friend, etc., but one with whom the daughter can establish a doctor/patient relationship in her own right, as proclaimed by one popular book title, *Our Bodies, Ourselves* (1976).

During early adolescent development, the pediatric model has advantages for both mother and daughter. It is familiar, comfortable, and does not threaten mother or daughter with the loss of closeness that comes with maturation. To the extent that the pediatrician has modified his practice routines so that he is practicing adolescent medicine with due regard for the developmental and psychological position of the teenagers, this modification would serve as a helpful transition to the adult-internist model. This is particularly so if he maintains a hovering flexibility of approach, leaning now more toward one paradigm, another time more toward the other, varying with his assessment of each situation and attuned fairly well to the needs of the daughter at that time.

However, at some point in the daughter's development, the pediatric model, even with its modifications and flexibility, has outlived its usefulness. At some point, the adult-internist model becomes a developmental necessity. The teenager who in absence of genital pathology uses the adult-internist model and obtains birth control/information demonstrates that she is the owner of her body, her self, and her genital, and has, to a great extent, relinquished her regressive relationship with her mother and her mother's fantasied ownership of

[7] I am aware that the daughter may often want her mother to know that she is sexually active and arrange for the mother to find out (such as in *Goodbye, Columbus*). However, I am emphasizing the possible breaks in confidentiality even when the desire to be discovered is minimal.

her genital. Thus, I propose that the teenager's seeking out of her own gynecologist on the adult-internist model is a progressive developmental step of great importance and as such is a behavioral manifestation[8] of the move from (re)discovery to ownership of the vagina.

I believe that ownership of the genital is an intermediary developmental stage in female sexual development which in too many instances *follows* chronologically the onset of sexual intercourse. From a contraceptive point of view, it would be desirable to have the ownership of the genital *precede* the onset of sexual intercourse. The question is whether the developmental line to ownership can be stimulated and ownership attained earlier—preferably before the onset of intercourse.

Admittedly speculative, I have the theoretical bias that the earlier use of the adult-internist model would be beneficial. Specifically, this can be initiated and/or offered to the adolescent girl by her mother, her pediatrician, or both. The most effective approach would for the mother to indicate to her daughter that when she is ready she can use the adult-internist model. Specifically, the mother should include the following points:

1. That she should have a gynecologist different from the mother's.

2. That the mother and/or mother's gynecologist could refer her to another gynecologist.

3. That she may and should call the gynecologist on her own when she finds it necessary, and that her mother will or will not accompany her, depending on the daughter's wishes.

4. That while the mother is interested to know and is available to be helpful, the mother grants her daughter the confidentiality and privacy of her own doctor/patient relationship.

5. That there may be questions and information she wants that she might not be able or want to discuss with her mother for which the gynecologist is available and can be useful.[9]

6. That specific organic pathology is not a prerequisite to a gynecologic consultation. In fact, it is preferable to have an initial visit in the absence of a specific complaint simply to get acquainted and get a baseline history.

7. That a pelvic examination would not be a requirement of such a "get-acquainted" visit, but a preparatory discussion and questioning could be useful.

[8]This is similar to the use of the menstrual tampon as the behavioral manifestation of (re)discovery mentioned in my earlier study (1979).
[9]These would probably be topics concerning birth control, venereal disease, masturbation, orgasm, and sexual dysfunction.

The fact that gynecologists with the requisite tact, manner, and knowledge of psychosexual female development are rare and often yet-to-be-trained is acknowledged. The educational effort which needs to be addressed with the gynecologist is perhaps in its embryonic state and worthy of the kind of extended commentary that would carry us beyond the limits of this chapter. My point is that such an effort is not a desirable and luxurious goal, but instead is a pressing necessity if the rising incidence of teenage pregnancy is to be reversed.

These same guidelines apply with obvious modification to the pediatrician, to indicate to the mother and her daughter that the latter is sufficiently mature to necessitate referral to a gynecologist. In fact, in some instances the pediatrician will have to take the initiative for such a referral, based on knowledge gained from either mother or daughter, or based on his or her perception that the mother's denial mechanisms are such that she minimizes her daughter's maturity, ignores the subtle but distinct messages of sexual interest and/or activity, and over-evaluates her daughter's "innocence" and abstinence. Again, the skill, knowledge, and perceptiveness of the average pediatrician may be wanting in this area; I wish only to emphasize the reasons and advantages for requiring and acquiring such pediatric skills.

SUMMARY

This chapter utilizes the concept of developmental lines leading to ownership of the genitals as applied to the problem of adolescent female nonuse of contraceptives. An intermediary stage of vaginal "(re)discovery" was delimited and defined in a previous communication (Shopper, 1979). The developmental line proceeding from vaginal (re)discovery to vaginal ownership involves genital sexual activity (masturbation and/or intercourse) as an intermediate facilitating activity. Yet, "ownership of the genital" is one of the developmental attainments necessary for the responsible utilization of contraception. If sexual intercourse is needed to attain "ownership," and "ownership" is needed to utilize responsible conception, then it follows that many adolescent girls will engage in sexual intercourse *before* utilizing adequate contraception. To the extent that this is true (to the extent that it is a dominant factor in an individual teenage girl), then greater availability of contraception, contraceptive information, and more and better sex education courses, as has been frequently recommended, will not have the impact hoped for by its proponents. The legal, epidemiologic, and cognitive approaches to contraceptive use must be supplemented by psychological measures which will (1) postpone sexual activity until there is more mature ego functioning, (2) enhance ego maturation in the area of vaginal "ownership," and (3) replace sexual intercourse with masturbation as an intermediate facilitating activity in the attainment of vaginal "ownership."

REFERENCES

Alan Guttmacher Institute. 1976. *11 Million Teenagers: What Can Be Done about the Epidemic of Adolescent Pregnancies in the United States.* New York: Planned Parenthood Federation of America.

Bergman, A. 1980. Ours, Yours, Mine. In R. Lax, S. Bach and J. A. Burland (Eds.): *Rapprochement, the Critical Subphase of Separation-Individuation.* New York: Jason Aronson, pp. 199–216.

Borowitz, G. H. 1973. The capacity to masturbate alone in adolescence. *Adol. Psychiatry* 2:130–143.

Boston Women's Health Book Collective. 1976. *Our Bodies, Ourselves.* Boston: Touchstone Books (Simon and Schuster).

Clower, V. L. 1975. Significance of masturbation in female sexual development and function. In I. M. Marcus and J. J. Francis (Eds.): *Masturbation from Infancy to Senescence.* New York : International University Press.

Goldsmith, S., Gabrielson, M. O., Gabrielson, I., Mathews, V. and Potts, L. 1972. Teenagers, sex and contraception. *Fam. Plann. Perspect.* 4:32–38.

Greenacre, P. 1958. Early physical determinants in the development of the sense of identity. *J. Am. Psychoanal. Assoc.* 6:612–627.

Kestenberg, J. 1961. Menarche. In S. Lorand and H. Schneer (Eds.): *Adolescents: Psychoanalytic Approach to Problems and Therapy.* New York: Paul Hoeber, pp. 19–50.

Kleeman, J. A. 1975. Genital self-stimulation in girls. In I. M. Marcus and J. J. Francis (Eds.): *Masturbation from Infancy to Senescence.* New York: Int. Univ. Press.

Laufer, M. 1968. The body image, the function of masturbation and adolescence: problems of the ownership of the body. *Psychoanal. Study Child* 23:114–137.

Lerner, H. E. 1976. Parental mislabeling of female genitals as a determinant of penis envy and learning inhibitions in women. *J. Am. Psychoanal. Assoc.* 24 (suppl):269–284.

Nadelson, C. C., Notman, M. T. and Gillon, J. 1978. Adolescent sexuality and pregnancy in the woman patient. In M. T. Notman and C. C. Nadelson (Eds.): *Sexual and Reproductive Aspects of Women's Health Care.* New York: Plenum.

Rennie, S., and Grimstead, K. 1975. *The New Woman's Survival Sourcebook.* New York: Alfred A. Knopf.

Rosenbaum, M. 1979. The changing body image of the adolescent girl. In M. Sugar (Ed.): *Female Adolescent Development.* New York: Brunner/Mazel, pp. 234–252.

Shah, F., Zelnik, M. and Kantner, J. F. 1975. Unprotected intercourse among unwed teenagers. *Fam. Plann. Perspect.* 7:32.

Shopper, M. 1967. Three as a symbol of the female genital and the role of differentiation. *Psychoanal. Q.* 36:410–417.

Shopper, M. 1979. The (re)discovery of the vagina and the importance of the menstrual tampon. In M. Sugar (Ed.): *Female Adolescent Development.* New York: Brunner/Mazel, pp. 214–233.

Winnicott, D. W. 1953. Transitional objects and transitional phenomena. In *Collected Papers: Through Paediatrics to Psychoanalysis.* New York: Basic Books, 1958, pp. 229–242.

4

The Psychodynamics of Teenage Pregnancy and Motherhood

SUSAN M. FISHER

This chapter could appropriately be subsumed under the broader topic, "The Vicissitudes of Adolescent Sexuality," or perhaps "The Development of Choice-Making Skills in Adolescents." I have narrowed the scope of inquiry. There is an increasing amount of high quality work being done on many phases of female adolescent development that covers the above noted dimensions (see Chapters 2 and 3, this volume).

The psychodynamics of teenage pregnancy cannot be seriously discussed in isolation from the backdrop of cultural differences and patterns of social class traditions and expectations. For each pregnant teenager, the meaning of her pregnancy will, of course, differ according to her own life story and individual family structure. Nonetheless, there are significant class differences in the handling and outcome of an adolescent pregnancy. For example, in Gardner and Fitchburg, Massachusetts, two heavily industrialized and working class towns, many of the pregnant teenagers come from families in which the mothers were also pregnant teenagers. In fact, the prime difference between mothers and daughters is that the younger group become pregnant two years before their mothers did. The highest teenage childbearing rates are in working class neighborhoods and depressed urban areas. In such towns, the pregnancy rate increases with the unemployment rate. These are communities where women have always married young; therefore, the generations are compressed. The notion of a pregnancy interrupting career plans is an unreal one, for most girls from these communities do not have a sense of a future career. It is important to remember that working class 16-year-olds who have babies are not dramatically worse off than their contemporaries without babies. For some girls, heretical as it seems, pregnancy can represent a thrust toward mastery and individuation. There may be vast feelings of inner emptiness; there may be intergenerational symbiotic conflicts; but one available route to economic independence can be a fatherless home with a child. Becoming pregnant may represent an attempt to grow up, an attempt that would have a different character for a middle class child.

Our appreciation of the psychodynamics of this complex phenomenon must, I think, be realistically based on the fact that there are whole sections of American society in which teenage pregnancy has been the norm for generations and will probably continue to be so. Stack (1974) suggested that for the displaced Southern black families she studied, having babies allowed the formation of kin ties and a method of recreating a stable community network in Northern towns.

Although there are some class differences in rates of pregnancy, the individual pathology may be the same for middle class and working class girls. The middle class families may push more actively for abortion. Middle class girls have a greater number of alternative channels to displace the same emptiness and emotional disturbance that may characterize all these girls, regardless of class. The same parent-child dynamic can hold in middle and working class girls, but sociocultural opportunities may make a delay of instinctual gratification via pregnancy and motherhood more tolerable for a middle class girl. The future-orientation allowed to middle class girls—college, lessons, a greater sense of economic hope—may not reflect genuine sublimations as much as a fortunate set of alternatives beyond pregnancy to deal with inner and outer conflicts.

Having alluded briefly to some of the class issues, I begin the discussion of dynamics with a somewhat pessimistic observation. Some girls are going to get pregnant not only because of complicated social reasons and the traditions of a particular subculture, but because they are responding to a peculiarly tenacious quality of the mother-daughter symbiosis. This symbiosis is very difficult to interrupt. A pregnancy may reflect a variety of overlapping psychodynamic issues for a teenage girl. It may represent an attempt to replace a lost object for the child or the mother; it may be an attempt to cure a mother's depression or an attempt to avoid separation; frequently there is an attempt to overcome early deprivation by identifying with the new baby as her own self. Sometimes, the newborn becomes a hostage to mother for the daughter's own subsequent liberation, with the daughter "free" to move on.

In my experience of supervising intensive outreach work in programs at Tufts New England Medical Center, I observed effective therapy on a 24-hour availability basis by street workers (called "anchor workers")—a one-person therapeutic environment. For some highly delinquent and depressed girls there was remarkable success in defusing explosive aggressive behavior, in improving self-esteem, in altering the quality of socialization, and in developing interests and skills that reflected some sublimations. But where there were severe early deficits in nurturance with a failure to stabilize an adequate self-concept, I frequently saw a compelling need to have a baby early. This dimension of character was most unresponsive to intervention. The pregnancy was sometimes understood to be a gift to mother, a bribe for the mother's hostility or mother's despair, an actual continuation of the tie to mother. But the forces that led to this need were so powerful and began so early that it was not an area of successful intervention. However, what significantly modifies this pessimism is that, regardless of the unconscious roots of her need to have this child, the outcome of the pregnancy, and the quality of sustained maternal care given the offspring, were deeply influenced by the other changes that had taken place in the girl. She was much more emotionally accessible to guidance by her worker. She wanted to be a good mother and all the various gains described above in impulse control, capacity to relate to others, and capacity to work were useful in her relationship with this baby.

CASE A

Kathy was one of a gang of girls who lived in abandoned cars, was involved in truancy and petty crime, spent a great deal of time in court, and was considered uncontrollable by family, courts, and juvenile workers. Much of her delinquent career was organized around attracting the attention of her withdrawn and rejecting mother and then punishing her. By age 17, after several years of contact with her street worker, she had graduated from high school with good grades and given up all delinquent activities. When she became pregnant, however, she considered no alternative to keeping the baby, but concentrated her efforts on becoming a good mother, using her worker as both a model and a source of guidance. She eventually married the child's father and took quite good care of her son.

This type of girl is severely disturbed. There are other girls who are less deeply troubled, who are amenable to briefer intervention. For these girls, pregnancy reflects an attempt to resolve an intense triadic conflict. Obviously for this group, there are also pregenital issues, as for the profoundly damaged ones there are always oedipal ones. The preponderance of oedipal issues make this group easier to treat. They are relatively rare, however.

CASE B

Martha's parents focused their disappointments in one another onto the fulfillment of their beautiful daughter. Their competition for her affections scarcely masked their disdain for one another. The father in particular had a highly eroticized relationship with her and was jealous and resentful of any boyfriends she had. When he came into her bedroom at night to talk he commented upon her face and figure excessively and sensually. The mother had never attempted to interrupt this tie. The relationship between mother and daughter had been adequate before puberty when mother "surrendered" the mantle of femininity to her exotic teenager. Martha's pregnancy disrupted the family in complex ways and her insistence on having and keeping the baby involved a large number of psychiatrists in her New England city. In treatment she was able to sort out many factors in her relationship to both parents and to her past and future. Eventually, she went back to college, married someone else, and raised her son quite adequately at last report.

Another group, different in character from the two described above, are the very young mothers, aged nine to fourteen. Pregnancy for this group is quite different than for the group aged 15 to 19. These "little girl" mothers constitute a very small group, with a very high proportion of abortions. For the very little girl the baby is often like a toy or cuddly creature representing at best a transitional object, or at worst a thing to be left in a corner. The issues for the girl aged nine to 14 usually revolve around very early problems with mothering. Frequently, there has been no fathering at all and a great longing for a father is present. The significance of absent fathering is often minimized in these girls. We can speculate on the impact of effective fathering: the affirmation of a girl's femininity that can make a delay of pregnancy more acceptable, or self-affirmation through pregnancy less necessary; the dilution or neutralization of hostile or ineffective mothering; the sense of a family life in which she is a child rather than a mother to her own mother.

CASE C

Randy was 12 when first evaluated by the team of therapists. Her mother was 13 when she was born and she has four younger siblings. She grew up in a household without men, a household dominated by her maternal grandmother and collateral female cousins, all women attempting to separate from maternal figures, and failing. She had no memories of her father or the other fathers of her siblings. She was thrown out of high school, and was heavily involved in vandalism. She repeated over and over the experiences of her mother. From childhood on she had a pattern of chronic, uncontrolled aggression. She was in a day hospital program where the danger of her becoming pregnant at the same age as her own mother had been thoroughly noted. Despite the therapeutic milieu and intensive individual therapy, she became pregnant at 13. Her mother took her for an abortion. She then ran away, overdosed in a rage at her mother, and continued the pattern of rage and aggression in an attempt to separate from her mother. The pattern of mutual destructive aggression between Randy and her mother that overlay the powerful symbiotic bond between them characterizes many of the girls in this very young group. The pregnancy and birth represent many aspects of this symbiotic tie and the attempts to breach it.

For the very young girl, the difficulty in her being pregnant is not simply her greater psychopathology, though that is frequently the case. These little girls have simply not experienced as much of life as older girls, experiences however conflictual and questionable that can become the matrix for later reworking and integration. If they deliver, these pubescent girls become mothers who can be shattered by the experience of pregnancy. Their body image is too inchoate to tolerate such a massive change. Their physiology is inadequate to handle the stress of pregnancy and they can suffer severe ego damage or developmental arrest. Recent studies (Baldwin and Cain, 1980) suggested that the health of the newborn child of a teenage mother is related to the quality of prenatal care; where the young mothers receive excellent care and nutrition, their babies are frequently healthier than the children of older mothers. For the mother below 14, however, the physiologic effects of a pregnancy and the psychologic impact on her own ego development are cause for alarm.

Baldwin and Cain (1980) pointed out that most earlier studies highlighted the relationship of the young age of the mother with increased risk of low-birthweight babies and perinatal infant mortality. The newer studies reveal that these phenomena are almost entirely related to the quality of prenatal care. That sounds an optimistic note indeed; however, they stressed that vigorous health at birth may be of short duration, for the subsequent health of her child may be severely jeopardized by early motherhood. Many analyses show deficits in the cognitive development of children, particularly males, born to teenagers (Baldwin and Cain, 1980). It is important to note, however, that the effect seems to result from the social and economic consequences of early childbearing.

The long-term followup of these children finds less consistent effects on social, emotional, and school development. These children are more likely to spend a considerable part of their development in one-parent households, and to have children as adolescents themselves. Research suggests that the children do best when raised in an extended family network where the teenage mother has help from her own family or the baby's father. The effect of mother's age on her child's social and emotional development does not appear to result from the mother's age per se, but is transmitted through the educational and economic disadvantages, greater likelihood of marital breakup, and the factors transmitted through the more difficult social context of the young mother.

Baldwin and Cain (1980) concluded their elaborate survey of the literature: "The research presented here suggests that one way to help the children of adolescents is to improve the education and employment opportunities of the teenage parents and to encourage the supporting role of other adult family members."

There are always many ways to subdivide or characterize a large cohort. My differentiation is based on a developmental perspective. There are three groups of pregnant teenagers that can be differentiated, with obvious overlaps between them.

First, the group of psychologically deprived, perhaps profoundly damaged girls for whom an infant fills a deep narcissistic need related to a faulty self-concept, to primitive object ties to the mother, and to powerful hungers for contact and affirmation. The subgroup of very young girls aged nine to 14 represents the group at the highest risk. Second are a group of better integrated girls attempting an oedipal resolution through pregnancy. Third is a group for whom pregnancy represents an attempt at maturation, an expression and substantiation of kin ties, the utilization of economic skills, a tradition of their group, a rite of passage.

The psychodynamics of teenage pregnancy may be usefully set against the changes in adolescence in the United States, where menarche occurs so much earlier and teenage life begins earlier and lasts longer. In many urban centers, teenage life begins at ten or 11 years. A generation ago, the years ten to 12 would show conventionally ascribed latency tasks in full bloom: hobbies, same-sexed peer friendships organized around activities, the pursuit of solitary pleasures of vast significance for the later self-discipline and aloneness that adult life requires, the strengthening of autonomous ego structures.

A corrective to the deprivations implicit in such a shortened latency has come from another change in teenage life. There is far more nonsexualized interacting among boys and girls as friends and persons, a shift in the character of adolescent object relationships that suggests a quality of relating reminiscent of latency. Sharing in groups coexists with relationships based on mutual sexual interest. These friendships provide a second chance for the foreshortened peer group experiences of latency.

The girl who becomes pregnant is prematurely and necessarily adult in her social focus. She is locked out of the gifts of latency by the culturally aborted premature adolescence experienced in the United States. Her pregnancy denies her this second chance to develop the ego resources that other adolescents can get from the peer group structure. What becomes arrested in these girls is the completion of the tasks of adolescence which for some may already have been difficult because of earlier conflicts and deprivations. By tasks, I mean the following irreducible human developmental issues that are not class-bound (Fisher and Scharf, 1980):

1. Nonsexualized socialization with a variety of peers, male and female;

2. The opportunity to regress in adolescence and thereby reexperience closeness and nurturance to gather strength for intimate relations at a more mature level;

3. The opportunity to rework the super-ego by opening up identifications

and testing boundaries—all in a more realistic manner, so that harsher, more magical super-ego structures are ameliorated;

4. The opportunity to develop skills and hobbies that further enhance autonomous ego functions to provide strength for disciplined tasks and the capacity for aloneness;

5. The making of career choices—the preparations for the nonlibidinal pleasures of adulthood;

6. Autonomous physical self-care.

The impulse to bear a child in the psychologically vulnerable girl is a very powerful one. To the extent that it is possible to interrupt that impulse, an effort is required in advance of a pregnancy to enhance the self-worth and self-esteem in a setting that will gratify the emotional needs basic to these girls and unfulfilled in them. Studies suggest that birth control information is not the answer, and that only ten percent of girls did not know enough to avoid pregnancy if they so wished, consciously or unconsciously. The setting that helps prevent pregnancy in the vulnerable girl is no different than the setting required to help the young pregnant woman. Anthropologic research (Fisher and Scharf, 1980) suggests that many non-Western cultures with early childbearing incorporate into their methods of child rearing and preparation for pregnancy these same characteristics of an effective setting. These characteristics are:*

1. It must provide a peer group of similar girls of the same age;

2. It must provide models of nurturance who nurture young mothers while showing them how to nurture their own babies;

3. It must provide models of admonition, rule-givers who gently discipline young childbearing clients when indicated and become models of limit-setting for the young;

4. It must provide structures to maintain and teach age-appropriate skills;

5. It must provide educational and career facilities for the further development of the childbearing girl;

6. It must provide adequate physical care for the pregnant girl and her baby;

7. It must recognize the role of the father, and acknowledge and involve him whenever possible;

8. It must continue services and client contact beyond the separation-individuation phase of the child.

Examples of programs that put into effect many of these characteristics can be found elsewhere in this volume. It is striking that many of the social problems encountered by teenage mothers in Western society are an exaggeration, even a caricature, of the problems of married adult mothers: the problems

---

*The author wishes to thank Dr. Roberta Apfel of Beth Israel Hospital, Boston, for her help in formulating these criteria.

of isolation, the lack of support and training for role change, and the deficiencies of extended networks of support. The problem is not just that these teenage girls are so inadequate and so young, it is that by being so young they are excluded from whatever support systems our society does provide.

It is the provision of those supports that can permit these girls to better mother this child born in their immaturity, and perhaps to grow as well in the process, and have less need to repeat premature pregnancies. Several programs have a remarkably low repeat rate. Programs attempting to respond to the needs of teenage mothers do best when they replicate what anthropology has discovered about those cultures which have pubertal mothers—an institutional or cultural pattern involving a combination of modeling, rule-giving and nurturance (Hagaman, 1977; Hart, 1965; Marshall, 1975; Mead and Bateson, 1954; Richards, 1961; Rubin, 1976). One could then, hopefully, satisfy the need for mothering in the pregnant teenager by using a mother substitute who can effectively meet the basic needs of the deficiently mothered girl, but in a form tolerable to the ambivalent adolescent who hates to acknowledge such needs. A more mature woman, more or less finished with adolescence, can ideally turn to her own mother for help. Having a child before the separation process is completed enormously complicates the normal regressive identifications that occur in pregnancy. The quest for an ego-ideal, part of normal adolescent development, exists in all these girls. The different role models available in successful programs present a range of such models in the external environment; these figures can nurture and educate these often inadequate psyches and be internalized as ego-ideal figures for the adolescent part of the self, and to ameliorate early developmental failures. In the proper setting, the state of openness and de-differentiation of ego boundaries that occurs during pregnancy and after delivery (Winnicott, 1958), with a temporary fluidity of defensive structure, can provide an opportunity for fruitful reworking, a second chance for these young mothers, in a setting similar to a "holding environment." It is clear that the best hope for the teenage mother, her baby, and any future children is a setting in which there are rich developmental possibilities for both mother and infant.

SUMMARY

I have attempted to integrate the individual psychology of the pregnant teenager, with all its complexity, into the social and cultural context of modern American life, with all its variations and changing character. Three developmentally diverse character structures are described. Some programmatic inferences are noted.

REFERENCES

Baldwin, W. and Cain, V. 1980. Children of teenage parents. *Fam. Plann. Perspect.* 12(1):34–43.

Fisher, S. and Scharf, K. R. 1980. Anthropological, psychological, and sociological overview of teenage pregnancy. *Adol. Psychiatry* 8:393–403.

Hagaman, B. 1977. *Beer and matriliny: The power of women in West African Society.* Unpublished dissertation. Northeastern University, Boston.

Hart, D. 1965. From pregnancy through birth in a Bisayan Filipino village. In D. Hart, P. Rajadhon, and R. Coughlin (Eds.): *Southeast Asian Birth Customs.* New Haven: Human Relations Area Files.

Marshall, J. 1975. *The Wasp's Nest.* Cambridge: DER Productions.

Mead, M. and Bateson, G. 1954. *Bathing babies in three cultures.* New York: New York University Films.

Richards, A. 1961. *Chisungu.* New York: Humanities Press.

Rubin, L. 1976. *Worlds of Pain.* New York: Basic Books.

Stack, C. 1974. *All Our Kin.* New York: Harper and Row.

Winnicott, D. W. 1958. *Primary maternal preoccuption.* In *Collected Papers.* London: Tavistock.

5

Boys Who Make Babies

JAMES M. HERZOG

By accident or by design, adolescent males father children. By trial or error, with greater or lesser success, some adolescent men parent their offspring. Little is known of the psychological determinants, internal or external, which account for either of the above-mentioned phenomena. Until recently, the whole area of male caretaking and its relationship to male sexuality was a relatively neglected and understudied area. A change is now occurring as fathers have been discovered—by themselves, by academicians, and by women's liberationists. A fairly consistent picture of the way in which fantasies, experiences, identifications, and interactions are forged into a nascent view of the self as provider and progenitor is beginning to emerge.

The connection between sexual behavior and caretaking is far from understood in adolescence. The rising adolescent birth rate, particularly in the face of widespread contraceptive availability, is particularly noteworthy. In those cases in which the father of the infant born to an adolescent mother is himself adolescent, is the conception and subsequent birth accidental or intentional? If intentional, whose intention does it reflect? The boy's, the girl's, the couple's, or someone else's entirely?

There are few systematic studies which address these issues. Furstenberg (1976) and the Offers (1974) have provided data on sexually active young men. The former study found 43 percent of males between the ages of 13 and 19 to be sexually active, whereas the latter reported only ten percent of males between 15 and 17 to be similarly engaged. The Furstenberg data is drawn primarily from an inner-city lower SES population, whereas the Offers' sample is derived from a more affluent middle class urban and suburban sample. A study by Jessor and Jessor (1977) suggested that females have a higher rate of sexual behavior during the junior and senior high school years than do males. They reported nonvirginity rates for females increasing from 26 to 55 percent. The corresponding rates for males went from 21 to 33 percent.

There is also some information about the variability in adolescent male sexuality among different ethnic groups. Finkel and Finkel (1975) reported that the mean age for first intercourse for white youth in New York City was 14.5 years; for Hispanic youth it was 12.8 years and for black youth it was 11.6 years. They also reported on contraceptive use in their study and seemed to find a difference along ethnic lines. It appeared that black and Hispanic youths not only become sexually active earlier but were less likely to use contraception— thus increasing the likelihood of conception.

Brunswick's (1969) study of Harlem youth suggested that many of her subjects did not give much thought to outcome events such as pregnancy or venereal disease, but rather were concerned with being able "to do it" and being in good shape. Brunswick also elicited information from her young subjects about their interest in marrying. For most of her 12 to 17-year-old respondents, marriage was anticipated in future decades rather than at the present time.

POPULATION AND DATA BASE

My own work with adolescent fathers has been in the context of studying male caretaking from a developmental perspective. In earlier work (Herzog, 1978) I suggested that the caretaking line of development in boys and men differs from that occurring in women. For men, a condensation of aggressive and libidinal components can be clearly identified at each stage and in suboptimal circumstances these constituent components can be seen to emerge with frightening clarity. I have also suggested that an ongoing heterosexual intimacy which permits expression, titration, and containment of sexual and aggressive drives seems to favor the emergence of optimal male caretaking (Herzog, 1980). This last concept has been stated rather succinctly as adult-adult interaction predicts adult-child interaction.

The clinical data which I shall present in this chapter derive from my leading four groups for junior and senior high school boys in an inner circle suburban high school over a four-year period in a nonclinical setting. The groups were billed as seminars in sexuality and intimacy. Corresponding groups for girls led by female mental health professionals were available simultaneously. Each group had eight to ten participants and met weekly for approximately thirty weeks. The participants in the groups corresponded to no particular diagnostic category nor was there a predominance of any particular character type. The dynamics of these groups were highly instructive. Transferential issues were very prominent as were issues of status and competition among the group members.

Information about the boy's sexual lives and practices emerged only slowly and in the context of growing familiarity, trust, and a group ethos. The manner in which this data emerged has raised many questions in my mind about personal sexual data obtained from adolescents by survey and questionnaire protocols.

From the data I have culled material pertaining to adolescent male caretaking from six of the boys. Since there were thirty-two boys who participated in the groups over the four-year period, this represents almost 20 percent of the group who were actively involved as 16, 17, and 18 year olds with issues directly related to male caretaking. I include in my sample young men who would not ordinarily be considered to be adolescent fathers. The reader will need to judge the wisdom or error implicit in these groupings.

In the first-year group, there were eight boys—white and middle class. Three pregnancies were reported during the year and all were to be terminated by abortion. This led to some discussion of the abortion experience. Matt, who was very involved with his girl friend Sharon and had been with her before and after the procedure, described a dream about Abraham sacrificing Isaac at the Lord's command. However, at the last moment the knife was plunged into Sarah, Isaac's mother. Matt commented on the fact that this was both the name of his girlfrield and the name of the Biblical Isaac's mother. One of the other group members, himself not yet the source of an abortus or other conceptus, told Matt not to take it so seriously—that it "was just a fluke" and wasn't it "nifty that a kid could be gotten rid of almost as quickly and easily as it could be made." At this point, Matt became very angry and then quite suddenly sad. He shared the fact that he had almost intentionally not used a rubber, that perhaps he had wanted to make Sharon pregnant—but he certainly didn't want to become a father.

Later when two other boys in the group impregnated more casual girlfriends and those pregnancies were to be aborted, the discussion came up again. "You win some, you lose some," was the prevalent group attitude. Matt challenged the two who were intensely involved in this—Jack and Joe—with, "How does it make you feel?" "Cocky," Jack answered with a grin. "Like handing out cigars," was Joe's reply. "You know, I sort of felt like a father or a father-to-be when Sharon was pregnant," Matt said. "But I couldn't imagine our having the kid, or taking care of him." The entire group of 16 and 17 years olds agreed that they didn't want to become fathers, yet a consensus emerged that it would mean something to make someone pregnant. This feeling coexisted with the feeling that the worst thing that could happen was to "knock someone up." There were jokes about shotgun weddings, irate fathers, and the law. The mood of the group was light-hearted and party-like until Matt recalled that Sharon cried sometimes when they talked about the abortion and that he sometimes felt that she didn't enjoy lovemaking now as much as before.

Then a rather startling occurrence was reported. Joe came to the group very shaken and reported that Liz, his casual paramour of some months earlier, had not had an abortion after all. He had happened to meet her and she was very visibly pregnant. Joe told us that he was very angry with Liz. She deceived him. Then he told us that he really hadn't had very much to do with her decision-making and certainly not with its implementation. Joe was clearly troubled. He developed a sleep disturbance and started to drink excessively. He asked if he could see me alone and then told me that he didn't know what he was feeling or what he should do. "There was really a kid inside Liz," "What should I feel about that?" He thought he hated Liz. But he couldn't just shrug it off. That kid was his, whatever that meant. He felt that he should do something, but he didn't know what. Then Joe, who was in some ways the most "macho" member of the group, began to cry. He expressed a strong wish that I contact his parents. He particularly wanted his father to know, but he felt afraid of his reaction. At the next group meeting, Joe told about his meeting with me. He said that he felt "all screwed up about this father" thing and that he had decided to go into psychotherapy. The reaction of the group was quite mixed. Matt was very supportive. Jack made a wisecrack to the effect that one paid his nickel and took his chance and then we moved on to other topics.

In another group, Brad told us that he was the father of two children, a boy of six months and a girl of nine months, and each one lived with its mother. Brad was friendly with each of the mothers, but had now fallen in love with Belle, a third girlfriend. Belle didn't want to get pregnant and Brad was relieved that she was on the pill. He said he certainly wasn't "going to wear anything or pull out early with a girl. You might as well use your own hand then." Brad told the group that he didn't see much of the kids now, but maybe he would when they got older. His mom kept in touch with the mothers of his two old girlfriends, the grandmothers of his son and daughter. "It sort of keeps it in the family," he said. The other boys in the group didn't know how to respond to Brad, but this was uniformly so, not only in regard to his attitudes toward fatherhood. Brad was from a different racial background than the other boys and was bused to the school from an adjacent part of the metropolitan area.

Two years later, Brad now almost 20, brought his now 2½-year-old son to a successor group. He seemed proud of little Sam and invested in him. When Sam knocked over another group member's books, Brad picked him up and gave him a spanking. This event resulted in a number of discussions among the group members on themes of anger, limit-setting, corporal punishment, and fathers. There ensued one of the most detailed discussions that had ever occurred about the boys' relationships with their own fathers, particularly with regard to discipline. At first there was a great embarrassment when the boys discussed lectures, spankings, and other punishments they had received. Later, this seemed to give way to camaraderie and backslapping. One of the boys wondered if I, the oldest male present and a father, was a spanker and if so, what kind. This question was followed by almost raucous laughter and speculations which ranged from my being the gentlest and most nurturant of men to my being a direct descendant of the Marquis de Sade.

Arthur was the quietest boy in his group. He spoke not a word as we talked about masturbation, intercourse, contraception, or venereal disease. There was general snickering when the topic of the day was homosexuality and Arthur developed a gastrointestinal disturbance and had to leave. When the topic was children, however, Arthur became more vocal. He shared with the group that he helped to care for Ricky, the two-year-old child of his unwed sister Jane, who lived in an adjacent neighborhood. Arthur saw Ricky and Jane on a daily basis. He babysat for his nephew and took him to the park. He reported that Ricky called him "Ar Ar" and told his Mommy that he "loved Ar Ar more than anyone else in the world." Arthur blushed as he told us that Ricky wanted to pee in the toilet just as he did and that his sister had told him that he, Arthur, was a wonderful father. When asked how he felt about Ricky, Arthur stated: "I love him." "It's good practice for you Art," one of the group members said. "Most of us don't get to practice being dads ahead of time."

Another group member, Frank, told us that he and Milly had been going together for a year and hoped to go to the same college to continue their close relationship. They hoped to marry after college and then, after law school, to have two children, hopefully a boy and a girl. Recently, Frank stated he and Milly had become intimate. Together, they had seen Milly's gynecologist, who also was their mothers' gynecologist. They had to be very certain to delay the arrival of Amanda and David, the names that they gave their future children. Both Frank's and Milly's families knew about the relationship but neither knew that a ten-year projection complete with grandchildren existed.

DISCUSSION

Matt, Jack, Joe, Brad, Arthur, and Frank are six young men, all of whom might be called adolescent fathers. Each boy's "fatherhood" was different. These experiences ranged from abortive to actual to substitutive to accidental to anticipatory. It seems that these cases tell us something, not only about the varieties of adolescent fatherhood that are encountered, but also something about the constituents, components, and conflicts characteristic of the male caretaking line of development during adolescence.

In thinking about fathering, we tend to think in terms of a series of functions: the way the father takes care of his child, the way he interacts with the child, the way he loves the child, the way he guides, teaches, and disciplines the child. Generally speaking, these activities are separated into discrete entities because they are then suitable for observation and study. In a naturalistic setting, it is highly probable that male caretaking is not emitted in discrete quanta of definable functions, although its inherent rhythmicity may be less tonic and more staccato than that characterizing female caretaking. Rather, there is a relationship between the male adult in the family and the children in the family which features both direct and mediated effects, substantially influenced by the adult female caretaker who is also present. That mother mothers, father fathers, and children develop in a context which is triadic at a minimum, is now a generally accepted point of view, even though it runs contrary to certain views of development which emphasize the essentially dyadic nature of early experience. We also know that parenting, both male and female, is an activity which grows better with practice. The very act of parenting seems to predispose to better parenting over time, provided of course that serious psychopathology is not present and exerting a deleterious effect on caretaking. Adolescent parents tend to have relationships of shorter duration than do older parents and by definition a shorter time experience of parenting than do older parents with multiple children. There is no data, however, to suggest that adolescent male parenting is different from that of older fathers. Kinard and Klerman (1980) and Bolton et al (1980) suggested that the incidence of abuse perpetrated by adolescent parents is no greater than that committed by older parents.

There is beginning to be observational data on what the business of fathering is, as distinct from mother. Parke (1981) in his book on fathering, reviewed the studies of Lamb, Clark-Stewart, Pederson, Yogman, Kotelchuk, and others, which demonstrated recognition of the father by the infant in the first months of life and an attachment relationship to him often as powerful as that occurring with the mother. In a study of eight middle class families consisting of a father, mother, and first child in the second year of life (neither parent an adolescent), I have detected some of the ways in which fathers, by virtue of being secondary rather than primary caretakers, appear to evolve a quite identifiable style of interaction and functional uniqueness with their children.

These interactions are often energizing, activating large motor activities which disrupt and delight the child. They appear to disorganize him in the sense of disturbing the status quo, and as such may mobilize intense affect which facilitates radical reorganization and further developmental progression. I have suggested that the radical reorganization-change of perspective paradigm may be the precursor to the quality which I have called ego resiliency and which may be a hallmark of children who are fathered as well as mothered.

This same mode of interaction—changing gears, jazzing things up, gross motor play—seems to be a modality by which fathers teach children not only how to mobilize drive and affect, but also how to modulate it. Within the play framework, and by departing from it, fathers model and express in more direct preverbal and verbal forms the range of expression of affect and action which they and their community will sanction.

It is very important to notice that these fathering functions can only occur in the presence of a mother. This kind of interaction with a child would be catastrophic if it were the only kind of interaction. The child would be driven to distraction in two hours if the only component of his developmental diet were stimulating, gear-shifting, disruptive, limit-setting play. The fathering I have been studying in the above-mentioned project is entirely contingent upon the presence of more homeostatic-attuned caregiving by the mother. In fact, male caretaking in a variety of settings seems to bear an important relationship to adult-adult male-female interaction. However, it should be noted that there are circumstances in which the male can become the primary caretaker. Then his style becomes more responsive and attuned. The father then comes to more closely resemble the homeostasis-maintaining maternal caretaker.

But what of the six boys whose experience with "fathering" I have reported on here? We know almost nothing of their actual interaction with their children since the only "observation" was of Brad with Sam, the only report was of Arthur with Ricky, and the only affective male-female relationships of Matt and Sharon and Frank and Milly did not involve an actual child.

On the basis of my data I cannot discuss the actual fathering of these young men. I can, however, advance some views on the meaning of the fathering concerns, plans, and fantasies of these six young men. My discussion will draw upon a nosology of the meaning of sexual behavior that I have developed.

I have classified sexual behavior according to its predominant meaning to the persons participating in it as declarative, recreative-interactive, procreative, parentogenic, and integrative. Of course, any sexual episode may contain elements of some or all of these meanings as well as a large admixture of more idiosyncratic meaning.

Declarative intercourse is "I am a man. I can do it." The partners' value need not be stressed and the empathy-intimacy dimension can vary from non-existent to profound. Recreative-interactive intercourse stresses the hedonic and social aspects of the act. Obviously, depending upon the particular dyad, one or the other pole of this form of intercourse may be stressed for the self or the partner. Procreative intercourse features the wish, often unconscious, to make a baby. It often also contains the opposite wish, to get rid of the baby once made. Parentogenic intercourse differs from procreative in that the wish to make a baby is coupled with the commitment to care for it. In my experience, parentogenic intercourse almost always occurs within the context of a relationship which features significant future orientation. Integrative sexual intercourse involves a feeling of oneness and wholeness with one's partner, a permeability of ego boundaries, and a resolution that leaves each participant feeling renewed and complete.

From a developmental perspective, it is not clear whether there is an intrinsic order to the aforementioned distinctions. In some ways it seems that a parentogenic and integrative sexuality corresponds to the later Eriksonian stages of generativity and integrity and might thus be considered a post youth-early adulthood phenomenon (1950). Declarative and recreative-interactive intercourse, on the other hand, appear to be the most common forms of masculine adolescent sexuality. Surprisingly, perhaps, I differentiate procreative (or conceptive) sexuality from a parentogenic sexuality. The former appears to exert considerable influence on adolescent masculine sexuality. Complicated forces from earlier developmental epochs appear to motivate the sexually active male to try to make a baby—to show that he can, that his stuff is adequate. For some boys, particularly those without other accomplishments, this seems necessary to maintain self-esteem. The procreative form of sexual activity sometimes also contains in quite clear view its opposite, the wish to get rid of or throw away the conceptus. This feature of male caretaking sometimes seems to contribute to instances of abuse and/or neglect. I have applied a similar scheme of categorization to adolescent female's sexual behavior.

In the examples which I have presented can be observed a wide range of reaction to the occurrence of an "unwanted" pregnancy. The nature of the relationship with the girl appears to impart the most important immediate component of the response, as with Matt. But, even the macho Joe reacted to "his baby," when an abortion did not occur. Joe's reaction is particularly significant because it did not seem to be relationship-dependent. Brad's experience tells us something about the different definitions of fatherhood which some cultural settings allow an adolescent male. Procreating and parenting are not necessarily closely linked temporally—but the right of fatherhood, once established, persists. Also, the father's role as modulator of aggressive drive and fantasy, often through the actual use of aggression, was clearly called forth by Brad's spanking of Sam and resonated with active currents of interest and concern in many of the boys. A theme of adolescent caretaking seems to be: can I do unto another what is still being done unto me. This permutation on the Golden Rule appears to apply to both libidinal and aggressive caretaking issues.

Arthur's experience seems to be an example of either preparing for parenthood or a situation in which massive psychological inhibitions favor the emergence of a substitutive behavior at the expense of more age-appropriate exploration and play. The number of adolescent males caring for children who are not their own is unknown. Clearly this is a very interesting group of young men for further study. A subgrouping of this category may be adolescent boys in fatherless families with younger siblings.

Frank's anticipatory fatherhood is equally intriguing. One cannot help but wonder if Amanda and David will ever arrive, how the discrepancy between what has so long been imagined and what actually occurs will be handled, and what the purpose of the decade-long gestational period really is. This is not to suggest that Frank's anticipatory fatherhood is abnormal. It is another variant of adolescent caretaking encountered in this setting.

None of the adolescent "fathers" described resembles the stereotype of the father in his late 20s, 30s, or 40s. Some may say that these boys were not actually fathers at all. By examining the experience of each of these boys, however, we may achieve greater clarity as to what fathering actually is and of what it is composed. The admixture of sexual development and meaning, of the capacity for intimacy and relationship, and of caretaking appears to be illuminated. As these men are in the earliest stages of their caretaking careers, we can perhaps more clearly appreciate the components, constituents, and conflicts which constitute the paternal posture.

SUMMARY

Experiences with groups of sexually active male adolescents are described. The varieties of paternal feelings, fantasies, and actualities encountered in these groups have led to a formulation about adolescent sexual and parental development. The study of these very early fathers will hopefully shed light on the caretaking line of development in both boys and men.

REFERENCES

Bolton, F. G., Lane, R. H. and Kane, S. P. 1980. Child maltreatment risk among adolescent mothers: a study of reported cases. *Am. J. Orthopsychiatry* 50(3):489-505.

Brunswick, A. 1969. Health needs of adolescents: how the adolescent sees them. *Am. J. Publ. Health* 59(9):1730-1745.

Finkel, M. and Finkel, D. 1975. Sexual and contraceptive knowledge, attitudes and behavior of male adolescents. *Fam. Plann. Perspect.* 7(6):256-260.

Furstenberg, F. 1976. *Unplanned Parenthood.* New York: Free Press

Herzog, J. M. 1978. *Patterns of Expectant Fatherhood.* Presented at the American Psychoanalytic Association Midwinter Meeting. New York, New York.

Herzog, J. M. 1980. *Adult-Adult Interaction Predicts Adult-Child Interaction.* Presented at the American Psychoanalytic Association Meeting. San Francisco, California.

Herzog, J. M. 1981. *Libidinal and Aggressive Availability, Aspects of the Father-Child Relationship in the 2nd Year of Life.* Presented to the 32nd International Psychoanalytical Congress. Helsinki, Finland.

Jessor, R. and Jessor, S. 1977. *Problem Behavior and Psychosocial Development: A Longitudinal Study of Youth.* New York: Academic Press.

Kinard, E. M. and Klerman, L. U. 1980. Teenage parenting and child abuse: are they related? *Am. J. Orthopsychiatry* 50(3):481-489.

Offer, D. and Offer, J. 1974. Normal adolescent males: the high school and college years. *J. Am. Coll. Health Assoc.* 22(2):209-215.

Parke, R. D. 1981. Fathers. In *The Developing Child Series.* Cambridge, Massachusetts: Harvard University Press.

6

The Role of Ethnic Factors in Adolescent Pregnancy and Motherhood

CARLOS SALGUERO

In the last decade significant attention has been given to the role of social, economic, psychological, and biological factors in adolescent pregnancy and motherhood. Study of population subgroups raises the question of their availability in public, welfare-funded clinics, hospitals, and health centers. Furstenberg's (1976) group of pregnant adolescents were very disadvantaged black adolescents. Other significant studies of teenage pregnancy (Battaglia et al, 1963; Klerman and Jekel, 1973; McAnarney et al, 1978; Spellacy et al, 1978) were of predominantly black populations.

Tietze (1977) found that white adolescents tend to have more abortions than black adolescents. Gutelius (1970) described the child-rearing attitudes of low income black adolescents.

In spite of these and other views of race as an important variable in adolescents' susceptibility to pregnancy and its outcome, there is a general consensus that it is so interrelated with socioeconomic conditions that race itself cannot be considered an independent variable for the determination of adolescent pregnancy or its effects on the adolescent during pregnancy and motherhood. For example, the National Center for Health Statistics (1980) reports that low birth weight among black babies continues to be much higher than among whites regardless of the age of the mother. This is partly because black women obtain prenatal care much later than white women.

Furthermore, most studies compare white populations with black or other nonwhite populations without recognizing trends observed in other significant ethnic groups.

This chapter compares seven variables among two different ethnic groups of adolescents—black and Hispanic*—who reside in an inner-city neighborhood of New Haven described in Chapter 11 (in this volume). The stimulus for the comparison of these two ethnic groups was the author's observation that although these two groups have socioeconomic characteristics similar to those in national populations, they are different with regard to their identity as mothers and in their attitude toward contraceptive practice and educational goals. The areas compared are the economic situation, family background, marital status, educational history, contraceptive practices, parity, and prenatal, birth, and delivery information. The data reported here are derived from the Hill Health Center's records of pregnant adolescents who went to term, and participated in the Teenage Pregnancy and Parenting Program (TAPPP) between November 1977 and July 1980.

The program was initiated in 1976 by the Mental Health Services Department of the Hill Health Center. The Center provides comprehensive services to 13,000 registered residents of the Hill neighborhood (population 24,000) of the City of New Haven. The Center is staffed by physicians (pediatricians, internists, obstetricians, child psychiatrists), nurses, dentists, nutritionists, community health workers, mental health specialists (psychologists, social workers, special education teachers), and support personnel and services. Hospital services are provided by the Yale-New Haven Hospital, six blocks away from the Center. In 1977, with funds provided by a demonstration grant received from the Administration of Children, Youth and Families, TAPPP expanded to coordinate services and assistance to sexually active and pregnant adolescents as well as young mothers and their children until the latter are 3.8 years old and can benefit from other state and federal programs. A primary worker, usually a social worker, follows the adolescent through pregnancy and early motherhood to provide her with practical and emotional support. TAPPP also has formal contacts with the school system and other community agencies who serve adolescents participating in our program.

Of the 78 pregnant adolescents in our TAPPP population for the year 1977-1978, 15 voluntarily aborted (Salguero et al, 1979). Of this abortion group, only one was Hispanic. The Hispanic adolescents' negative attitude towards abortion is based on their concept of motherhood and womanhood. Hispanic adolescents tend to leave their home and live with their mates at a younger age than black adolescents and are expected to bear children to show

---

*In this chapter the term *Hispanic* designates those adolescents who have a Spanish surname and either they and/or their parents came from Puerto Rico.

independence. However ambivalent they feel about the pregnancy, abortion, especially in the younger-aged Hispanic group, is not considered an alternative outcome. But, we have observed a sharp increase in the number of therapeutic abortions in the group aged 18 and over.

DATA BASE

In the present study, data were obtained from Hill Health Center records of 86 adolescents—29 Hispanics and 57 blacks—who were followed by TAPPP continuously from November 1977 to July 1980, all of whom delivered during this period. However, data are not uniformly complete for all adolescents, with more information being available for those who delivered early in the project and remained in our program than for those who delivered late in the period or moved out of the catchment area. In some cases, the data collection effort was hindered by the unwillingness of some adolescents to discuss their relationship to the baby's father, especially if he was not involved with the adolescent. Since it is a voluntary program, no specific data were requested of the adolescents and the information emerged through their spontaneous interactions with TAPPP staff. The information presented here, however, is significant enough in the areas considered for appropriate comparisons between the two groups. The clinical observations about the adolescents are drawn from the TAPPP worker's assessment of the adolescent, her family, and circumstances. Servici (1979) statistically established the credibility of reports and observations made by Hill Health Center social workers in their work with adolescent mothers.

Economic Situation

Table 1 shows the source of income for both groups. Welfare dependency is the main source of financial support, with 65 percent (56 of 86) receiving

Table 1. Support Source of 86 Black and Hispanic Adolescents at Time of Conception

Source	Black		Hispanic		Total	
	N	%	N	%	N	%
Welfare	39	68	17	59	56	65
Work	12	21	6	21	18	21
Both	3	5	3	10	6	7
Other	2	4	3	10	5	6
Not known	1	2	0	0	1	1
Total	57	100	29	100	86	100

Table 2. Distribution of 86 Black and Hispanic Adolescents' Living Situations
During Pregnancy, Three Months, and One Year After Delivery

Living Situation	Black (57)		Hispanic (29)		Total	
	N	%	N	%	N	%
During pregnancy						
Living with own family	54	95	14	48	68	79
Living on her own	0	0	1	3	1	1
Living with partner	0	0	11	39	11	13
Other	3	5	3	10	6	7
Total	57	100	29	100	86	100
Three months after delivery						
Living with own family	49	86	8	28	57	66
Living on her own	3	5	4	14	7	9
Living with partner	3	5	16	55	19	22
Other	0	0	0	0	0	0
No information	2	4	1	3	3	3
Total	57	100	29	100	86	100
One year after delivery						
Living with own family	28	49	4	14	32	37
Living on her own	10	18	4	14	14	16
Living with partner	7	12	13	45	20	23
Other	0	0	7	24	7	9
No information	12	21	1	3	13	15
Total	57	100	29	100	86	100

welfare assistance at the time they became pregnant. This figure increases to 72 percent (62 of 86) if one takes into account those families in which a member of the family or a partner worked while the rest of the family received welfare support. Twenty-one percent (18 of 86) of the adolescents came from working families. Hispanic adolescents over 16 years of age who left home after getting pregnant became primary welfare recipients after delivery, initiating a new cycle of welfare dependency.

Family Background

At the time the adolescents became pregnant and during their pregnancy, 68 of the 86 lived with their families of origin (Table 2).* For the black population, this accounted for 95 percent (54 of 57). Thirteen of 54 black adolescents

*Data throughout this chapter have not been examined to offer statistical significance or correlational values.

living with their families came from intact families. The remaining adolescents lived in a one-parent family. With few exceptions, the adolescent's mother was the head of the household. Of the other siblings living in the family home, at least one was close to the adolescent's age and also at potential risk for pregnancy. Three months after delivery, only five of the 54 black adolescents had moved away from home. From then on, there was a gradual shift towards socioeconomic independence by young black mothers. Yet, one year after delivery, 28 or almost 50 percent of these mothers still lived with their families while ten lived on their own and seven lived with their partner.

In comparison, only 14 of the 29 Hispanic adolescents (48 percent) lived with their family of origin after becoming pregnant. Of these, only four came from a two-parent family. In most cases, the family was made up of the adolescent's mother, siblings, and other extended family members. Eleven adolescents lived with their partner during pregnancy. Three months after delivery, only 28 percent (eight of 29) of these Hispanic mothers lived with their family, while 55 percent (16 of 29) lived with their partners. This trend continued after one year with more mothers establishing their own lives alone or with a partner.

Marital Status

Although most of the group of 86 adolescents were single, it is noteworthy that, with one exception, all black adolescents were single, but eight Hispanic girls were married during their pregnancy (Table 3). There was a trend for the male Hispanic partner to be much older and therefore expecting a marital relationship. For these adolescents the choice of living with, and getting pregnant by, an older person is not accidental. Elements of security and some marital stability enter into the contract.

Table 4 shows that the Hispanic group of male conceptual partners tended to be older than the black group.

Table 3. Marital Status of 86 Black and Hispanic Adolescents During Pregnancy

Status	Black (57)		Hispanics (29)		Total (86)	
	N	%	N	%	N	%
Single	56	98	21	72	77	90
Married	1	2	8	28	9	10
					86	100

Table 4. Comparison of Black and Hispanic Adolescents' Partner's Ages
at Time of Conception

Age	Black (57)		Hispanic (29)		Total (86)	
	N	%	N	%	N	%
14–17	10	18	2	7	12	14
18–21	23	40	7	24	30	35
22–25	4	7	11	38	15	18
26–29	1	2	1	3	2	2
30+	1	2	2	7	3	3
No information	18	32	6	21	24	28
Total	57	100	29	100	86	100

The degree of involvement with, and support given by, the male partners to the pregnant adolescents and their offspring was observed by our staff. The degree of commitment was determined by our staff from observations based on the presence or absence of the father during a clinic visit made by the adolescent, his interactions with her and the baby at home and at the clinic, and the adolescent's comments about him. Highly committed partners were perceived as caring and helpful to the adolescent girl and her child. They often helped financially, babysat, and came to the clinic with the young mother and her baby; many of them lived together. For purposes of classification, the staff viewed the partner's commitment as excellent, good, fair, or poor. Some partners had no relationship to the female partner or baby. In 19 cases, the staff were not able to ascertain the partner's age. The topic of boyfriends was particularly sensitive and uncomfortable for the adolescents. In some cases, the baby's father disengaged himself from the relationship with her or joined the armed forces, or the adolescent felt this was a private matter she did not want to discuss with staff. Our continuous relationship did give us an idea, however, of the male partner's involvement. Living together, as in the case of the Hispanic partner, did not mean that the mates were more supportive than cases in which this was not the case (Table 5).

In some cases, the relationship between the adolescent girls and their partners changed over time. This may have been due to our better understanding of the young mothers' relationships to their mates. Less than one third of the pregnant adolescents and young mothers in the black group had an "excellent" relationship with their boyfriends while roughly another third had a "poor" relationship before and after delivery.

This relationship did not change much at one year after delivery. In the Hispanic group the number of partners who had an "excellent" commitment

Table 5. Black and Hispanic Adolescents' Partners:
Commitment Status During Pregnancy and Subsequent to Delivery

Commitment	Black (57)	Hispanic (29)	Total (86)
During pregnancy			
Excellent	14	8	22
Good	9	5	14
Fair	9	5	14
Poor	18	9	27
Unknown	7	2	9
Total	57	29	86
Three months after delivery			
Excellent	14	2	16
Good	6	8	14
Fair	10	8	18
Poor	17	10	27
Unknown	10	1	11
Total	57	29	86
One year after delivery			
Excellent	9	3	12
Good	8	7	15
Fair	5	5	10
Poor	16	8	24
Unknown	19	6	25
Total	57	29	86

to their girlfriends decreased, from eight during pregnancy, to three at one year after delivery. The numbers of those who had a "poor" relationship did not change much over the period of time considered.

Educational History

Table 6 shows that most of the adolescent girls in both groups became pregnant during or seen after they completed the ninth grade. Hispanic adolescents become pregnant while in lower grades than black adolescents. This finding is significant since many Hispanic adolescent girls drop out in the transition from junior high to high school or soon after they start high school. They may also be academically retarded compared with black age-mates even though intellectually there is no difference.

Table 7 shows the distribution of adolescents who remained in school, in another special program, or at home. Seventy-seven percent (44 of 57) of the black adolescents remained in school after getting pregnant, while 17 percent

Table 6. Comparison of Black and Hispanic Adolescents'
Educational Level at Time of Conception

Grade	Black (57)	Hispanic (29)	Total (86)
5	0	1	1
6	0	1	1
7	1	0	1
8	6	11	17
9	18	12	30
10	13	3	16
11	14	1	15
12	5		5

(five of 29) of the Hispanic adolescents remained in school. The number of
Hispanics remaining home after delivery—83 percent (24 of 29)—is overwhelming. The data show that in spite of the multiple demands pregnancy makes on
the adolescent, the black adolescent, when compared with her Hispanic counterpart, makes better use of the family and community supports to continue in
school before and after delivery. At one year after delivery, almost 50 percent

Table 7. School-Work-Home Situation Status of Black and Hispanic
Adolescents During Pregnancy After Delivery and One Year After Delivery

Situation	Black (57)	Hispanics (29)	Total (86)
During pregnancy			
At school			
Junior High	5	1	6
High School	39	4	43
Working	1	1	2
Home	10	20	30
Other	2	3	5
No information	0	0	0
After delivery			
At school	33	2	35
Working	2	2	4
Home	21	24	45
No information	1	1	2
One year after delivery			
At school	27	2	29
Working	2	2	4
Home	14	18	32
No information	14	7	21

Table 8.   Contraceptive Use at Time of First Conception Among
Black and Hispanic Adolescents

	Black (57)		Hispanic (29)		Total (86)	
	N	%	N	%	N	%
Using birth control	15	26	1	4	16	18
IUD	4	7	0	0	4	4
Condom	1	2	0	0	1	1
Foam	1	2	0	0	1	1
Pill	9	15	1	4	10	12
No information	5	9			5	6
Not using birth control	37	64	28	96	65	76

(27 of 57) continued in school while 62 percent (18 of 29) of the Hispanics remained at home. As the boyfriend of one Hispanic adolescent put it when asked about the girl returning to school after having her baby, "Going back to school? Man, she is a mother, she's got plenty of things to do around the house."

Contraceptive Practices

Table 8 illustrates contraceptive practices for these adolescents before conception. Only those adolescents for whom the medical chart indicated that a form of birth control was prescribed before conception were listed as using birth control. Thirteen black adolescents and only one Hispanic adolescent had a documented history of using birth control. The vast majority of adolescents—76 percent (68 of 86)—denied ever using any method of birth control or claimed use of a contraceptive prescribed by another hospital or clinic, which often was impossible to document. Although readily available, contraceptives were inconsistently used by adolescents except for those pregnancies that occurred with an intrauterine device. It is possible that more than one Hispanic adolescent had used some artificial method of birth control, despite the positive cultural significance that virginity has for the Hispanic woman. Clinical experience has shown that many Hispanic men do not favor the use of birth control by their female mates in the belief that she will not be loyal to him. Thus, the apprehension about birth control by women in this group and the fact that they live with a man makes them quite vulnerable to subsequent pregnancies.

Parity

Table 9 illustrates parity and age at time of first and subsequent delivery for both groups. The majority of the black adolescents (61 percent, 35 of 57) delivered for the first time at age sixteen and seventeen. Twenty-six percent

Table 9. Parity and Age at Time of First and Subsequent Delivery
for 57 Black and 29 Hispanic Adolescents

Age	First Delivery Black (57)	First Delivery Hispanic (29)	Second Delivery Black (15)	Second Delivery Hispanic (11)	Third Delivery Black (2)	Third Delivery Hispanic (4)	Fourth Delivery Black (0)	Fourth Delivery Hispanic (1)
13	1							
14	3	2	1					
15	8	9						
16	17	10	1	3				
17	18	6	4	7				
18	10	2	5	1	1	2		
19			3			2		1
20			1		1			

(15 of 57) of the adolescents in the black group had another pregnancy in adolescence at a mean age of sixteen years and four months. By comparison, the majority of Hispanic adolescents (65 percent, 19 of 29) delivered for the first time when they were fifteen and sixteen years of age. Thirty-eight percent (11 of 29) of the Hispanic adolescents had another teen pregnancy at a mean age of fifteen years and seven months. In addition, the Hispanic adolescents in this subgroup had more third pregnancies (four) than the black subgroup. One young Hispanic mother had her fourth child at nineteen.

The median time elapsed between first delivery and second pregnancy was seven months for black mothers and 8.5 months for Hispanic mothers (Table 10). It is well known that the impact of a second pregnancy makes it even more difficult, if not impossible, for young mothers to meet their own social, educational, and emotional needs. These young mothers, especially in the Hispanic group, settle into a maternal role for which they are most often ill prepared.

Prenatal History, Birth, and Delivery Information

The Hill Health Center and TAPPP with its emphasis on community outreach have influenced the prenatal care patterns of adolescents participating in our program. Table 11 indicates that ten percent (nine of 86) of our population started receiving prenatal care during the third trimester of pregnancy. Fewer blacks (five percent) started their care during the third trimester than Hispanics (21 percent).

The quality of prenatal care is similarly distributed (Table 12), with 57 percent (49 of 86) of the adolescents receiving excellent prenatal care. Our staff considers prenatal care to be excellent, when the adolescent has eight or more prenatal visits; fair, if five to seven visits; and poor, for less than five visits, or if the adolescent starts prenatal care in the third trimester.

The gestational age at the time of delivery was estimated by Hill Health Center obstetricians by dates, clinical examinations, and ultrasonograms. Seventy-three percent (63 of 86) of the infants had a gestational age of 38 to 40 weeks at delivery, and only 13 percent (11 of 86) were 35 to 37 weeks (Table 13).

There were no significant differences between the two groups in regard to labor and delivery data. Eighty percent (69) had a normal vaginal delivery while 11 percent (10) had a Caesarean section, seven due to cephalopelvic disproportion and three due to failure of labor to progress. The number of maternal complications during labor and delivery was not surprisingly high for adolescents, with 33 percent (19 of 57) and 28 percent (eight of 29) for blacks and Hispanics, respectively. The most frequent problems were high blood pressure, anemia, and toxemia (see Chapter 7, this volume). The number of adolescents experiencing complications is not high enough to show a statistically significant difference between the two groups. Proportionately, however, four black adolescents and only one Hispanic adolescent had anemia serious enough to warrant treatment at the time of delivery. The incidence of toxemia was low for both groups (six percent) when compared with the 15 percent reported for other groups (Alan Guttmacher Institute, 1981). The birth complications were surprisingly fewer than expected, with only one birth complication in the Hispanic group. Only one infant weighed less than 4 lbs at birth. The mean birth weight was 6 lb 10 oz for blacks and 6 lb 4 oz for Hispanics.

DISCUSSION

A review of the seven trends for each ethnic group illustrates the similarities and differences between them. Black and Hispanic adolescents resided in the Hill neighborhood and were therefore exposed to the same social pathology observed in the catchment area, that is, a high incidence of unemployment, crowded housing, crime, and drugs. The majority of the girls came from one-parent families who were receiving welfare assistance. Often there were other siblings at home who already had young children or were at risk for pregnancy. The girls were noncompliant contraceptors and became pregnant on average at age 15.5 years. There were no significant differences between these groups in relation to age at time of conception.

The health patterns of both groups also followed similar trends with a higher number in both groups starting their prenatal care in the first trimester of pregnancy (53 percent) than in the other two trimesters. As a result, both groups also experienced maternal complications during labor and delivery but to a lesser degree than reported by Clark (1971) and Magrab and Danielson-Murphy (1979). These infants had an unusually low incidence of prematurity, birth

Table 10. Time Elapsed Between Previous Delivery and Subsequent Impregnation for 15 Black and 11 Hispanic Adolescents

Recidivist Black Adolescent Subject No.	Age at First Delivery	Age at Second Delivery	Age at Third Delivery	Age at Fourth Delivery	Time Elapsed* (in months)
1	16 yrs 8 mos	18 yrs 2 mos			9
2	13 yrs 5 mos	14 yrs 9 mos			7
3	18 yrs 0 mos	20 yrs 1 mos			16
4	17 yrs 3 mos	19 yrs 5 mos			17
5	15 yrs 7 mos	16 yrs 6 mos			2
6	15 yrs 5 mos	16 yrs 5 mos			3
7	16 yrs 1 mos	17 yrs 4 mos			6
8	18 yrs 4 mos	19 yrs 5 mos			4
9	16 yrs 7 mos.	18 yrs 0 mos			8
10	16 yrs 9 mos	18 yrs 4 mos	19 yrs 5 mos		10
11	17 yrs 2 mos	18 yrs 7 mos			8
12	16 yrs 0 mos	17 yrs 1 mos	18 yrs 3 mos		4
13	16 yrs 11 mos	17 yrs 8 mos			0
14	16 yrs 0 mos	17 yrs 1 mos			4
15	16 yrs 6 mos	18 yrs 1 mos	20 yrs 0 mos		10

Median elapsed time between first delivery and second impregnation for Blacks = seven months.

Recidivist
Hispanic Adolescent
Subject No.

Subject No.					
1	16 yrs 0 mos	17 yrs 9 mos			12
2	16 yrs 1 mos	17 yrs 6 mos			8
3	15 yrs 5 mos	18 yrs 0 mos			22
4	15 yrs 9 mos	17 yrs 9 mos	18 yrs 10 mos		15
5	16 yrs 0 mos	16 yrs 11 mos			2
6	15 yrs 10 mos	17 yrs 6 mos	18 yrs 6 mos	19 yrs 9 mos	11
7	16 yrs 5 mos	17 yrs 10 mos	19 yrs 1 mos		8
8	15 yrs 1 mos	16 yrs 7 mos			9
9	15 yrs 9 mos	16 yrs 9 mos			3
10	15 yrs 3 mos	17 yrs 8 mos	19 yrs 6 mos		9
11	15 yrs 10 mos	17 yrs 1 mos			6

Median elapsed time between first delivery and second impregnation for Hispanics = 8.5 months.

*Time elapsed between delivery and subsequent impregnation was determined by subtracting nine months from the number of months between each delivery.

Analysis: Use median time to minimize effect of outliers in the data.

88　　　　　　　　　　　　　　　　　　　　　　　　　Carlos Salguero

Table 11.　Distribution of Black and Hispanic Adolescents by Trimester
of Prenatal Care Initiation

Trimester	Black (57)	Hispanic (29)	Total (86)
First	33	13	46
Second	21	10	31
Third	3	6	9

complications, and infant deaths during the first year of life, when compared
with other adolescent groups reported by the Guttmacher Institute (1981).
According to that Institute's latest report, improved prenatal care has reduced
prematurity and low birth weight among all age groups, but mothers aged 15 and
younger are still twice as likely to have low birth-weight babies when compared
with mothers aged 20 to 24. Among all teenagers, the risk for prematurity is
about 39 percent higher than for adults.

When each group was examined separately, both black and Hispanic
girls had a number of characteristics in each of the areas considered, from which
a profile for each group emerged which may have significant preventive
implications.

PROFILE OF THE BLACK ADOLESCENT MOTHER

The data show that the black adolescent came from a one-parent family in
which the mother was the main provider. This girl was approximately 15.8 years
old, single, and attending the ninth grade when she became pregnant for the first

Table 12.　Distribution of Black and Hispanic Adolescents
by Prenatal Care Rating*

Quality	Black (57)		Hispanic (29)		Total (86)	
	N	%	N	%	N	%
Excellent	36	63	13	45	49	57
Fair	12	21	9	31	21	24
Poor	9	16	7	24	16	19
Total	57	100	29	100	86	100

*Quality Scale
Excellent = eight prenatal visits or more
Fair = five to seven visits
Poor = less than five visits or only third trimester care.

Table 13. Labor and Delivery Information for Black and Hispanic Adolescents

Gestational Age (Weeks)	Black (57)	Hispanic (29)	Total (86)
≤ 34	0	1	1
35–37	9	2	11
38–40	40	23	63
≥ 41	5	3	8
No information	3	0	3
Type of delivery			
Normal vaginal delivery	45	24	69
Caesarean section	7	3	10
Forceps	3	1	4
Vacuum	0	1	1
No information	2	0	2
Maternal complications			
None	34	21	65
High blood pressure	6	4	10
Anemia	4	1	5
Toxemia	4	2	6
Other	5	1	6
No information	4	0	4
Birth complications			
None	51	28	79
Complications	5	1	6
No information	1	0	1
Birth weight (lbs)			
≤ 4	1	0	1
4–4.15	0	3*	3
5–5.15	5	6	11
6–6.15	27	7	34
7–7.15	20	6	26
8–8.15	5	5	10
9–9.15	0	3	3

*Twins.

time. She had been using some form of birth control inconsistently and was not using it at the time of conception. Zelnick and Kantner (1980) reported that the average age at which black adolescents initiate intercourse is 15.5 years. Zabin et al (1979) also reported that 50 percent of all teenage pregnancies follow within six months of the adolescent's first sexual experience. Thus, the black adolescents in our sample are similar to those groups of sexually active black adolescents.

The black adolescent continued to live with her family throughout her pregnancy. Our staff often felt that however inadequate the family support, it was her main economic and emotional support which made it possible for her to continue school during pregnancy and after delivery. When the young mother felt more comfortable in her new role and adjusted to a new image of herself, she moved out to her own apartment or to live with her boyfriend. As Lorie, a seventeen-year-old said, "It was time for me to move and try it out on my own."

The black adolescents' boyfriends were young men in their late teens or slightly younger, who, when committed to a long-term relationship, provided some emotional support. Often they were unemployed and remained home with the baby while the adolescent mother went to school; or, they visited the mother and baby. Many young men often terminated their relationship with the girl after she became pregnant. One out of every three known partners was considered to have a "poor" relationship to his girlfriend (32 percent) during her pregnancy. This figure remained the same one year after delivery.

Pregnancy finds the young boyfriend as emotionally unprepared as the girl. Although peer group pressure plays a role in encouraging pregnancy, the black adolescent male in our sample had enough awareness of the significance of having a child of his own to continue a positive relationship of varying degree with his girlfriend during pregnancy (57 percent). This commitment decreased to 52 percent at three months after delivery and 37 percent at one year after delivery. In the author's opinion this is not a discouraging figure, given the emotional and maturational adjustment these young partners have to make to continue a more permanent and meaningful relationship with their girlfriends and babies.

From data not included in the tables, we find that at one year after delivery a slight majority of black adolescents in our sample were not attending school (down to 47 percent from 58 percent attending three months after delivery). Factors such as moving from her mother's home and inadequate baby-sitting arrangements were responsible for this drop in school attendance. Nevertheless, she had not become pregnant a second time. For those who had a second child (26 percent), the elapsed time between the birth of the first child and the new pregnancy was seven months, a comparatively low figure. Jekel et al (1973) reported 30 percent of 73 poor school attenders were pregnant again by 15 months. In Klein's (1974) sample of 1,824 adolescents aged 16 years of age or under, 10.7 percent had a repeat second pregnancy; of these, 41.9 percent became pregnant within a year after the first delivery.

Among the factors (other than ethnicity) that play a role in the black adolescent's pregnancy outcome, especially in regard to her return to school, are the degree of family support and attainment of gradual independence and self-competence. The TAPPP extensive medical and social outreach, with its close links to the school system and other community agencies, seems to have affected all these areas, although other influences cannot be denied. Furstenberg and Crawford (1978) reported that of those young mothers who lived with parents or relatives, 87 percent remained in school after childbirth compared with 76 percent of those who lived alone, and 60 percent got jobs compared with 41 percent of those who lived alone. Thus, the black adolescent's success in some of the tasks of adolescence, such as to complete education, become independent, and gradually view herself as a mother, is determined by a commitment, however ill-defined, by her family to her well-being and to her bettering herself.

PROFILE OF THE HISPANIC ADOLESCENT MOTHER

The Hispanic adolescent has a different profile than her black counterpart. Our data found her to be approximately 15.5 to 16 years of age, about to enter high school or in the ninth grade, and in the process of leaving her family of origin at the time of conception. In 39 percent of cases she was living with her partner. I have observed that with the advent of adolescence there is a shift in the relationship of the Hispanic girl with her mother. The mother now ceases nurturing and pampering and views her daughter's efforts towards independence with apprehension since she fears she will lose her virginity soon, become pregnant, and follow the mother's fate.

Padilla and Ruiz (1973) described the general structure and function of Mexican-American and Puerto Rican families, especially the submissive role of the mother in the family: "Ideally women are perceived as sexually pure, but pragmatically, they are seen as generally defenseless and particularly vulnerable to seduction by the sexually attractive and powerful Puerto Rican male. These husbands and fathers expect women to respond with passive compliance."

Such behavior, imprinted since childhood, is viewed as a desirable attribute which defines her as unselfish, maternal, and dedicated to her children and home in emulation of the Virgin Mary. Stevens (1973) calls, "marianismo" that constellation of attributes which enables women to bear the indignities inflicted upon them by men and to forgive those who bring them pain. Protecting the virginity of their adolescent daughters is part of the family honor and the sexual purity expected of these women. It is not uncommon for mothers to ask the obstetrician at the health center about her daughter's virginity. According to Abad et al (1976), "Virginity is highly valued by the Puerto Rican woman. She is taught to be submissive and obedient to men and may well experience conflict with Anglo values on the mainland." They stated that adolescent girls may seek to be more assertive and independent like their Anglo peers and in doing so risk alienation from their parents and their cultural group. Thus, the Hispanic adolescent in her efforts to develop more autonomy, soon becomes involved with a man, usually in his mid-20s or older. The relationship between daughter and mother is tenuous enough that the Hispanic adolescent moves to her own or her partner's family apartment with her partner and assumes the role of common-law wife.

Our data show the Hispanic girl to be a noncompliant contraceptor. Most of the reasons given by Hispanic girls to TAPPP staff are, "The pill is bad for you," or "He'll (my boyfriend) think I'm cheating." One out of four Hispanic girls in our sample was married to her partner. As Anita, an 18-year-old Hispanic mother of two, said, "You want to marry somebody old so they don't cheat on you, but they do it anyway."

The motivation for the Hispanic adolescent to continue in school is very poor. The lack of incentive to view school realistically as a positive experience and her own sexual turmoil account for her dropping out. Once she is committed to a relationship with a man who views her as a partner who is expected to be home, since she will be a mother, it is impossible for her to attend school. Efforts by our staff to help Hispanic adolescents remain in school have been fruitless. The delivery of her own child established the adolescent, in the eyes of her family and her partner, as a mother and woman in her own right.

Although there is a definite shift towards physical separation from her family, daughters often move only a few houses away from their family of origin. There is now an egalitarian mother-daughter relationship which allows the Hispanic adolescent and her mother to relate to each other positively. Return to school is now next to impossible. When I suggested that Shelly, a 17-year-old, return to school, her partner said, "School? She is a mother, she's gotta look after the baby." Except for those Hispanic adolescents who exhibit signs of social psychopathology and whose infants are at high risk for abuse and neglect (Salguero et al, 1980), it has been observed that the young Hispanic mother finds fulfillment in remaining at home with her infant and finds a great deal of support and help from her mother, siblings, and other family members.

Since very few Hispanic adolescents use birth control after delivery, they have a greater risk of a second pregnancy. The elapsed time between delivery and her second impregnation was 8.5 months. By the time the Hispanic adolescent is 19 and pregnant for a third time, it is very likely that she will request a tubal ligation after delivery.

The Hispanic male of our sample is similar to the one described by Abad et al (1976). He is usually unemployed, through lack of education and training skills, or holds a temporary unskilled job. He may be supportive of his female partner during pregnancy. This support gradually wanes after delivery so that at one year after, the relationship is "poor" or he no longer lives with her. Thus, it is not surprising, as we indicated earlier, that only very few Hispanic adolescents come from an intact family. We do not have data on motives (bilaterally) for arrangements in living together of young girls and young boys versus older men. To maintain a positive image of himself, the Hispanic male relies on "machismo" behaviors, which at best is an unstable defense against castration anxiety. It has been described as a desirable combination of virtues, courage, and fearlessness in a man, which when threatened, leads to acting out behavior in drinking and sex (Aramoni, 1972; Abad and Suarez, 1975).

Ethnic factors cannot, by themselves, be responsible for adolescent pregnancy, but they do play a role in the meaning a pregnancy has within that person's cultural context. Just as blacks are very conscious of their blackness, its meaning, and its roots, so are Hispanics conscious of their background, regardless of class and educational status. Comer (Kolansky, 1981), reflecting on his years as a college student, stated that "though achievement and recognition in high school had been my way of being black, now my blackness became evident." Similarly, Butts (1979), in discussing the characteristics of black adolescent sexuality, believes that the black child learns early what it feels like to be black. She added that "the concept of race is the lesson to be learned first and foremost in the black child's socialization process." The black population considered in this chapter share some of these commonly held cultural values, especially the support that the black adolescent's family provides for her and other children (Davis, 1968). This commitment by the black family also reflects a better assimilation of blacks into the mainstream of American society and its values. This process of assimilation has been a lengthy and painful one to be sure. It has met with prejudice and discrimination since the days of slavery (Spurlock and Lawrence, 1979). According to Bettelheim and Janowitz (1964), signs of significant improvement in the social status of blacks began in the 1930s with the development of trade unions which unionized unorganized workers and thereby changed the socioeconomic status of blacks. From World War II to the present, improved employment opportunities, legal changes, the mass media, and an era of economic prosperity decreased racial prejudice and allowed blacks to have greater participation and say in American society via political parties, community organizations, and social groups. As a result, blacks have greater upward social mobility than before and better access to social, educational, and economic benefits. This does not mean, however, that the black adolescents in our sample and their families live in excellent conditions. Poverty, unemployment, and social pathology were found in many homes. In some cases, the TAPPP worker found the father absent or in jail, while an alcoholic mother looked after her adolescent daughter's children while the latter attended school. In other cases, the grandmother kicked her granddaughter out of the house for being defiant. But as Comer (personal communication, 1978) correctly points out, ". . . this has nothing to do with being black."

In conclusion, the majority of black adolescents in our sample availed themselves of health, social, and educational services offered by community agencies. This was possible because they had the basic family support necessary to help them deal with the system more effectively.

The majority of Hispanic adolescents in our sample were born in Puerto Rico. As an ethnic group (Knutson, 1965) they practice those values given to them by their culture through their family and have a common cultural identity. They have brought with them distinctive cultural traditions, customs, beliefs, and practices. The acceptance of other American ways does not lead to a disregard of long-held cultural traditions which may concern matters of modesty, taste, attitudes towards medicine, family structure, social and sexual behavior, or even the ways of using alcohol and expressing pain. The Hispanic families in our catchment area form a subculture, in which they put into practice those values that seem to give a logical meaning to their daily life via their contacts with other people at church, the "Hispanic-American" grocery store, or at the health center, to name a few areas of contact. This attachment to their values provided them with a sense of security, especially when the Anglo system is viewed as impersonal and uncaring. Many of these values clash with values held by the mainstream of American society and are not fully understood by Americans. For example, since the attainment of motherhood is highly valued by Puerto Ricans and other Spanish-speaking groups (Fernandez-Marina et al, 1958; Diaz-Guerrero, 1955), the male partner views his mate as a woman, wife, and mother and not as a teenager going back to school after having a baby. Her mother also holds this expectation; as a result, the young Hispanic mother will remain home. This is in contrast to the black grandmother who helps her daughter return to school. Ghali (1977) correctly stated that the machismo of the male and the marianismo of the female are roles that are looked down upon by Anglos. A Puerto Rican mother, concerned about her daughter's virginity, will be derogatorily accused of being overprotective and old-fashioned. According to Martinez (1979), Hispanic boys and girls find themselves in an educational system that offers very little in terms of realistic education or preparation for life. Martinez quoted a New York city social worker who told him that ". . . they all get wasted. The boys don't know what to do with themselves and neither do the girls. They end up trapped into playing house and inevitably the girls get pregnant. . . ."

The Hispanic adolescent female growing up in this environment finds herself attending a school where she is exposed to values which conflict with her own. Lacking her family's guidance and commitment to deal with the challenges and problems posed by the school system, she drops out and soon gets pregnant. By adhering to her family values, the Hispanic adolescent further distances herself from the values of mainstream American society which prevents her from finishing her education and improving her social and economic situation. The more isolated the Hispanic family is from the other elements of society, the more it entrenches itself in isolationist behaviors. The Social Science Research Seminar on Acculturation (1954) noted that forced acculturation thwarts creativity, unsettles traditional controls, fosters intergenerational and other conflicts, and may lead to cultural disintegration as manifested by a neglect of ceremonial observances, a dependency relationship with the dominant group, and, according to Favazza (1980), diminished physical and mental health. In the case of the Hispanic population from our catchment area, they do not have the community support necessary to develop new ways of thinking to achieve the internal adjustments necessary before accepting other values or redefining their own. Canino and Canino (1980) state that the Puerto Rican family has often borne not only the stress of migration but, along with other low-income Americans, the various strains of poverty: limited education, low income, discrimination, depressed social status, deteriorated housing, and minimal political influence.

CONCLUSIONS

A population of black and Hispanic adolescent mothers was studied and compared on seven variables. The most significant difference noted was the ability of many of the young black mothers to return to school while their Hispanic counterparts dropped out of school when they became pregnant. We believe that certain cultural values held by the two groups account for the different profiles described for the black and the Hispanic adolescent. Although no one factor explains why adolescents get pregnant, each ethnic group fared differently. In our opinion, the values held by each group do play a role in pregnancy outcome.

This is a report on a small group of black and Hispanic adolescents who became pregnant and delivered. The findings, therefore, cannot be generalized to other groups. It is clear that much additional work will be required to enlarge our understanding of how each ethnic group copes with the demands of early motherhood. Whether differences or similarities exist, it is agreed that both groups need a great deal of support by the different community agencies that serve them. Both groups are very deprived socioeconomically and face many obstacles in establishing their own identity. Both groups are at risk for being prematurely thrown into a mothering role for which they are ill prepared.

The TAPP Program is especially concerned about the school drop-out group who lack follow-up by the school system. The task of the school system, as that societal agency that educates and promotes growth and development without discrimination, will be a challenging one in implementing creative programs for adolescents, whether they have entered the stage of parenthood or not. Such programs should be sensitive to the cultural background and life circumstances the adolescent faces. Grandmothers should be invited to the classroom to share their mothering experiences, and fathers to discuss their own sense of family values and attitudes. All of these approaches should be blended into educational parenting techniques which may help young mothers and fathers become better parents who can recognize their infants' needs, and who can promote, as Anastasiow suggests (Chapter 10, this volume), normal child growth and development. It is through learning and education that adolescents will develop a better future orientation and better sense of themselves whether they go to college or become parents. As Fisher and Scharf (1980) stated, some girls are going to get pregnant no matter how extensive the intervention and prevention, not only because of complex social and traditional subcultural reasons, but because of the peculiarly tenacious quality of the symbiosis within the maternal line.

In addition to the school, other community agencies such as colleges universities, community centers, hospitals, health centers, churches, and the arts, to mention a few, should take more responsibility to better ethnic relations and improve minority education. Through our intensive outreach, we are learning more about the adolescent's family, and by providing them with support and assistance we are trying to prevent its further alienation from the community. We have found most of these families to be receptive and willing to share their concerns and needs. We believe that it is the system's turn to help them with respect for their values and traditions.

SUMMARY

This chapter compared seven variables in two ethnic minority groups of adolescent mothers—black and Hispanic. The variables are economic, family background, marital status, education, contraception, parity, and prenatal, birth, and delivery data. The data indicate that while black adolescent mothers are gradually being assimilated into mainstream American society, the Hispanics are isolated from it. Recommendations are given to prevent further alienation from the community while respecting their values and traditions.

ACKNOWLEDGMENTS

This work was supported by Grant 90-C-1337 from the Administration for Children, Youth and Families. The author thanks Ms. Renee Dinkins for assistance in data collection for this chapter.

REFERENCES

Abad, B., Ramos, J. and Boyce, E. 1976. A model delivery of mental health services to Spanish speaking minorities. *Am. J. Orthopsychiatry* 44:585–596.

Abad, V. and Suarez, J. 1975. *Cross-cultural aspects of alcoholism among Puerto Ricans.* Proceedings of the Fourth Annual Alcoholism Conference of the National Institute of Alcohol Abuse and Alcoholism. DHEW Publication No. 76-284: 282–294.

The Alan Guttmacher Institute. 1981. *Teenage Pregnancy: The Problem that Hasn't Gone Away.* New York.

Aramoni, A. 1972. Machismo. *Psychology Today* 5:69–72.

Battaglia, F., Frazier, T. and Helleger, A. 1963. Obstetric and pediatric complications of juvenile pregnancy. *Pediatrics* 32:902–910.

Bettelheim, B. and Janowitz, M. 1964. *Social Change and Prejudice.* New York: Free Press.

Butts, D. J. 1979. *Adolescent Sexuality and The Impact of Teenage Pregnancy from a Black Perspective.* Family Impact Seminar, George Washington University, Washington, DC.

Canino, I. A. and Canino, G. 1980. Impact of stress on the Puerto Rican family: treatment considerations. *Am. J. Orthopsychiatry* 50:535–541.

Clark, J. 1971. Adolescent obstetrics: obstetric and sociologic implications. *Clin. Obstet. Gynecol.* 14:1026–1036.

Davis, E. B. 1968. The American Negro: family membership to personal and social identity. *J. Natl. Med. Assoc.* 60:92–99.

Diaz-Guerrero, R. 1955. Neurosis and the Mexican family structure. *Am. J. Psychiatry* 112:411–417.

Favazza, A. 1980. Culture change and mental health. *J. Operat. Psychiatry* 11(2): 101–119.

Fernandez-Marina, R., Maldonado-Sierra, E. and Trent, R. 1958. Three basic themes in Mexican and Puerto Rican family values. *J. Soc. Psychol.* 48: 167–181.

Fisher, S. and Scharf, K. 1980. Teenage pregnancy: an anthropological, sociological and psychological view. *Adol. Psychiatry* 8:393–403.

Furstenberg, F. 1976. *Unplanned Parenthood: The Social Consequences of Teenage Childbearing.* New York: McMillan.

Furstenberg, F. and Crawford, A. 1978. Family support: helping teenage parents to cope. *Fam. Plann. Perspect.* 10:322–333.

Ghali, B. S. 1977. Culture sensitivity and the Puerto Rican client. *Soc. Casework* 58:459–468.

Gutelius, N. 1970. Child-rearing attitudes of teenage Negro girls. *Am. J. Publ. Health* 60:93–104.

Jekel, J., Klerman, L. and Bancroft, R. 1973. Factors associated with rapid subsequent pregnancies among school-age mothers. *Am. J. Publ. Health* 65: 370–374.

Klerman, L. and Jekel, J. 1973. *School Age Mothers: Problems, Programs and Policy.* Hamden, Connecticut: The Shoe String Press.

Klein, L. 1974. Early teenage pregnancy, contraception and repeat pregnancy. *Am. J. Obstet. Gynecol.* 120:249–256.

Knutson, A. 1965. *The Individual, Society and Health Behavior.* New York: Russel Sage Foundation.

Kolansky, E. Interview with James P. Comer, M.D. *Am. Acad. Child Psychiatry* Newsletter, Spring 1981. Washington, D.C.

Magrab, D. and Danielson-Murphy, J. 1979. Adolescent pregnancy. A review. *J. Clin. Child Psychol.* 8:121–125.

Martinez, L. A. 1979. *Adolescent Pregnancy: The Impact on Hispanic Adolescents and Their Families.* Family Impact Seminar, George Washington University, Washington, DC.

McArnaney, E., Roghmann, E., Adams, B., Tatalbaum, R., Kash, C. and Coulter, M. 1978. Obstetric, neonatal, and psychosocial outcome of pregnant adolescents. *Pediatrics* 61:199–206.

National Center for Health Statistics. DHHS (NCHS). 1980. Final Natality Statistics, 1978. *Monthly Vital Statistics Report.* 29:1–27.

Padilla, A. and Ruiz, R. 1973. *Latino Mental Health, A Review of the Literature.* DHEW Publication No. (ADM) 76-113. Washington, DC: U.S. Government Printing Office.

Salguero, C. Suarez, J., Yearwood, E. and Schlesinger, N. 1979. *Report: Teenage Pregnancy and Parenting Program.* New Haven, Connecticut: Hill Health Center.

Salguero, C., Yearwood, E., Phillips, E. and Schlesinger, N. 1980. Studies of infants at risk and their adolescent mothers. *Adol. Psychiatry* 8:404–421.

Servici, I. 1979. *Adolescent Pregnancy at the Hill Health Center: Factors Predicting Infant Development in the First Year of Life.* Medical School Dissertation. New Haven, Connecticut: Yale University School of Medicine.

The Social Science Research Council Summer Seminar on Acculturation. 1954. Acculturation: an exploratory formulation. *Am. Anthropol.* 56:973–1002.

Spellacy, W., Mahan, C. and Cruz, A. 1978. The adolescent's first pregnancy: a controlled study. *South Med. J.* 71:768–771.

Spurlock, J. and Lawrence, L. E. 1979. The Black Child. In J. Noshspitz (Ed.): *Basic Handbook of Child Psychiatry.* New York: Basic Books.

Stevens, E. 1973. Machismo and marianismo. *Society* 3:57–63. New Brunswick, New Jersey: Rutgers State University.

Tietze, C. 1977. Legal abortion in the United States: rates and ratios by race and age. *Fam. Plann. Perspect.* 9:12–15.

Zabin, L., Kantner, J. and Zelnick, M. 1979. The risk of adolescent pregnancy in the first months of intercourse. *Fam. Plann. Perspect.* 11:215–222.

Zelnick, M. and Kantner, J. 1980. Sexual activity, contraceptive use and pregnancy among metropolitan-area teenagers. 1971–1979. *Fam. Plann. Perspect.* 12:230–237.

The Infant—
Developmental Risks

7

Infants of Adolescent Mothers: Research Perspectives

MAX SUGAR

With the increased incidence of baby-keeping by adolescent mothers, it is important to consider whether and how this increases risks to the infant. Since most
adolescent mothers are unwed, the effects of father absence on the infant also
become significant. The physical and emotional readiness of adolescents to be
pregnant and become mothers are different from those of adults. Relevant
research is reviewed and the results of single unwed motherhood and an absent
father on their youngsters' development are detailed.

SCOPE OF THE PROBLEM

Currently, in the United States alone, there are over three million live
births a year. Approximately 600,000 of these births are to teenagers in the 15-
to 19-year-old age group. Annually, 30,000 unmarried girls under the age of 14
become pregnant. Eighty-five to 95 percent of teenage mothers now keep their
illegitimate children, while 18 percent of white and two percent of black illegitimate children are given up (Zelnick and Kantner, 1974).

This is not an isolated phenomenon limited to the United States. A recent
report from Yugoslavia (Beric et al, 1978) detailed the increase in adolescent
pregnancies and illegal and legal abortions. Katz et al (1977), in a review of
pregnancy in the unwed, white South African found, that 78 percent of the
English-speaking girls kept their babies. Eighty-three percent used no contraception and eight percent were totally ignorant of contraception. By comparison,

61 percent of Afrikaans-speaking girls kept their babies, 87 percent used no contraception, and, of this group of mothers, 18 percent were totally ignorant of contraception.

In 1971, in the United States, 52 percent of premaritally pregnant whites were married before the outcome of their pregnancy in contrast to 36 percent in 1976. The whites were four times more likely to marry before delivery than blacks. In the study, fewer than a fourth of the pregnant adolescents intended to become pregnant. Among those who did not intend pregnancy and used some birth control method, the rate of contraceptive use decreased from 17 percent in 1971 to eight percent in 1976 (Zelnick and Kantner, 1978).

One of the features requiring consideration is the earlier onset of menarche in the United States, which has dropped since 1900 from a mean of 14.2 years to 12.8 years in 1960, and to an estimated 12.5 or 11.8 at present (Cutright, 1972). In males, the average age of nocturnal emission is now estimated to be 12.2 years of age (Eskin, 1977). This indicates that both male and female partners are capable of activity leading to conception much earlier than in the past. By contrast, a study in New Guinea of the population of Sepik River natives found menarche (mean) to be 18.4 years. Sepik young people ordinarily marry a few years after that and birth of the first child occurs at a mean age of 23 years. The authors (Sturt and Sturt, 1974) compared this with Australia, Japan, and Costa Rica, where the respective mean ages for first childbirth are 23, 26, and 21 years. Reasons for the earlier menarche in the United States are unclear.

Low socioeconomic backgrounds have usually been connected with the higher risk of teenage pregnancy as well as a higher risk of complications for the pregnant adolescent, the adolescent mother, and her infant. These girls tend to have their first baby early in life (age ten to 15) and they produce more babies (eight to ten) than the average woman. They also continue to have children beyond the normal childbearing age (Anastasiow et al, 1978).

New York City data show that 73 percent of black families there are at high risk, as well as 38 percent of Puerto Rican families. Thirty percent of all births are illegitimate; among blacks the rate is 2.5 times that of white girls of the same age, and the highest rate (75 percent) is in Harlem. National statistics from 1966 to 1973 indicated that the birth rate has decreased 29 percent for 18 to 19 year olds and the illegitimacy rate has decreased 27 percent during the same time. However, the birth rate for 11 to 13 year olds increased 29 percent and the illegitimacy rate increased 47 percent for this same age group during these years (Kihss, 1977).

ADOLESCENT PREGNANCY RISKS AND EFFECTS

What are the risks to the infant of an adolescent mother? Let us divide this into a three-fold view: first, the effects of being a pregnant adolescent and its effect on the infant; second, the effects of not having a husband during her

Table 1. Comparison of Crises in Pregnancies of Adolescent
and Adult Mothers by Infants' Birth Weight

Infants	Birth weight (g)	Crisis in:		X^2	df	p*
		Adolescent mother N (percent)	Adult mother N (percent)			
Premature	≤2,500	161 (56.5)	160 (35.6)	12.33	2	0.002
Full-term	≥2,501	53 (55.7)	107 (33.6)	8.41	1	0.004
All infants		214 (56.3)	267 (35.2)	20.74	3	< 0.001

*If p <0.05, the percentages are significantly different.

pregnancy and motherhood nor a father for the infant; and third, the combined effect of all these factors on the infant and its subsequent development.

During adolescent pregnancy, according to various surveys, 50 to 80 percent of the girls relate that they do not want the pregnancy. Therefore, there is less likelihood of normal preparatory thinking or fantasizing about the anticipated baby. The adolescent continues with conflictual thoughts since she has marked ambivalence about having the baby versus having an abortion, giving up the baby, or keeping it.

In my study (Sugar, 1979) of the pregnancies of 481 adolescent and adult mothers, the adolescent mothers of premature infants had a 57 percent rate of crisis in pregnancy compared with 36 percent for the adult mothers of prematures. Adolescent mothers of full-term infants had a 56 percent crisis rate versus a 34 percent rate for the adult mothers of full-terms. For all the infants, premature and full-term, adolescent mothers had a 56 percent rate of crisis compared with a 35 percent rate of crisis for the adult mothers. Among the mothers of prematures (birthweight less than 2,500 g), 52 percent were 19 years of age or younger while among mothers of full-term infants there were 33 percent who were 19 years or younger (Table 1).

Genetic studies indicate a high rate for Down's syndrome for the infants of mothers who are under 15; this equals the rate for women of 35 (Erickson, 1978). There is also a higher risk in young mothers of translocation Down's syndrome. The rate of risk to siblings of this translocation from a carrier parent increases to the younger mother under age 30, who has a rate of 83 percent, whereas the woman over thirty has a 1.9 percent translocation syndrome rate (Mikkelson, 1967).

The national prematurity rate is about eight percent, that is, about a quarter of a million infants annually in the United States are born prematurely. In a special program at Yale University, Jekel and associates (1975) found that among adolescent girls there was a 12 percent rate of prematurity but adolescent controls had a 27 percent premature birth rate. The risk of perinatal mortality for the infant born while the mother was in the program was two percent; however, when the mother was not in the program it was nine percent. Thirty-two percent of the low birthweight infants died when the mothers were not in the program, whereas none of the low birth-weight infants died when the mother was in it.

They further noted that there is a specificity related to birth order for the children of adolescent mothers. The perinatal death rate was less than one percent for her first child, seven percent for her second child, and 14 percent for her third child. The prematurity rate similarly climbed from 11 percent for the first infant to 21 percent with the second and 43 percent with the third. Adolescent mothers not in this special program had fewer prenatal visits and their offspring had an even higher rate of prematurity and perinatal death. Waters (1969) similarly found a 23 percent prematurity rate for subsequent deliveries to adolescent mothers beyond the first infant.

Erkan et al (1971) found a 50 percent preeclampsia rate in the 12-year-old mother and a total rate of 14 percent for the 12- to 15-year-old mothers. Their group of 14-year-old mothers had a 34 percent prematurity rate, and the overall rate for the adolescent mothers was 23 percent. If the mother became pregnant within two years of menarche, the mother had a 31 percent premature birth rate and a 19 percent preeclampsia rate; if the mother had her first baby two years or more after her menarche, she had a 16 percent prematurity rate and an 11 percent preeclampsia rate. The adolescent has a higher mortality rate during pregnancy and delivery, a higher rate of complications of pregnancy, such as toxemia, and a higher perinatal morbidity rate than the adult mother. Ruppersberg (1973) noted that adolescents constituted nine percent of the maternal death rate; 37 percent had an infant who weighed 2,500 gm or less, and only 49 percent had live births. (Fifty-one percent resulted in abortion, miscarriage, stillbirth, or dead adolescent.)

Adolescents as a group are prone to use and abuse chemical substances, among which are marijhuana, LSD, PCP, cigarettes, and alcohol. The effects of these on pregnancy and the fetus are unclear except for smoking and alcohol. Cigarette smoking contributes to a lower birth weight (Lowe, 1959; Simpson, 1957). Excessive alcohol intake in pregnancy may result in particular patterns of congenital anomalies and low birthweight, called the fetal alcohol syndrome. These include cardiac septal defects, genital abnormalities, hemangiomas, as well as behavioral, limb, craniofacial, and neurologic abnormalities. Those affected have an IQ of 35 to 40 points below normal (Hanson et al, 1976; Jones and Smith, 1973, 1975; National Institute on Alcohol Abuse and Alcoholism, 1977).

Toxemia and prematurity interfere with the mother's involvement with her infant due to their immediate separation, as is also the case when the baby is born by Caesarean section. What are some of the effects of the mother-infant separation? Early contact for 45 minutes immediately postpartally with the mother is significant for the infant's development and for the mother's involvement, with demonstrable effects at 12 and 36 hours (Hales et al, 1975, 1977). The mothers with the extended contact with the infant (consisting of an additional 16 hours in the first three days) picked up their babies more frequently one month postpartum in response to crying, had a greater tendency to stay home with their infants, were more comforting in stressful office visits, and showed more fondling and increased eye-to-eye contact.

At one year, extended-contact mothers showed distinct positive differences in their behavior and involvement with the infant compared with the control mothers (Kennell et al, 1974). In a study of the speech patterns of extended-contact mothers and their infants at age two years, the mothers used significantly more questions, adjectives, words per proposition, and fewer commands in content words than the control mothers. They had a distinctly greater variety and elaboration of verbal output than the control mothers, and used more appropriate forms of imparting information, for eliciting responses from the child and for elaborating simple concepts (Ringler et al, 1975).

In a follow-up study at age five years, the children who had extra contact with their mothers postpartally had higher IQ scores and a better understanding of complex phrases than the control children (Ringler et al, 1978).

Smith and associates (1975) found that by carefully scrutinizing the actual caretaking of infants of adolescent mothers, only seven percent actually cared for their infant even if they stated that the infant was under their care.

In my study (Sugar, 1979), the mother's knowledge of her infant's day-to-day behavior and development in the first six months was tabulated. These included her visiting frequency during the nursery stay; onset of finger and thumb-sucking, cooing, two-hand-eye coordination, recognition of mother's voice and face, exogenous smile, sitting, teething, eating, sleep, excretory, and play patterns; methods she used for managing these things; and the infant's involvement with those around it. An uninvolved mother does not know these things and her limited knowledge reflects deficient maternal bonding. Even if the infant is getting adequate care by another caretaking person, the intimate details are not known to the mother. A scale derived from this involvement was used to assess indirectly the adequacy of the mother's stimulation of her infant.

As shown in Table 2, the percentage of adequate stimulation by adolescent versus adult mothers of the premature infants was 73 and 85 percent. For full-term infants, adequate involvement was provided by 84 percent of adolescent mothers versus 89 percent of adult mothers. Contributions to the adolescent mother's inadequate stimulation appeared to be her narcissism, inadequate

Table 2. Comparison of Adequate Stimulation of Infant
by Mother's Age and Infant's Birth Weight

Infants	Birth weight (g)	Adolescent mother N (percent)	Adult mother N (percent)	X^2	df	p*
		Adequate Stimulation by:				
Premature	≤2,500	160 (73.4)	161 (85.2)	6.72	2	0.035
Full-term	≥2,501	53 (83.6)	107 (94.3)	4.38	1	0.036
All infants		214 (76.3)	267 (89.4)	11.10	3	0.011

*If p <0.05, the percentages are significantly different.

preparation for motherhood, neonatal deprivation (since most of the premature infants had a lengthy hospitalization), and divided mothering.

Inexperienced, primiparous mothers take longer to feed their infants, change their feeding activity more often, and stimulate their infants more than multiparous mothers do. Yet the infants of primiparous mothers consume less if they are bottle-fed and suck less if breast-fed than infants of multiparous mothers. Differences in sucking patterns were not apparent when infants were fed by an experienced nurse (Thoman, 1975).

Collingwood and Alberman (1979) reported a significantly higher proportion of rejected index children (RIC) than either non-rejected index children (NRIC) or control mothers under age 20 years and a significantly lower proportion of RIC (two of six) than NRIC (22 of 26) mothers aged from 20 to 34 years at birth of their study children (p = 0.02). A greater proportion of RIC than NRIC or control mothers were in the youngest age group (15 to 19 years) at time of giving birth to their first child.

Brown and Bakeman (1977), in studying predictors of maternal involvement with prematures at nine months, observed that education is the best single predictor. The infant's condition at birth is the best predictor of maternal involvement if maternal education and persistence are controlled.

EFFECTS OF FATHER PRESENCE

In white families in the United States, father's absence changed from eight to nine percent from 1950 to 1972, while father absence of all ages increased in nonwhite families from 18 percent in 1950 to 30 percent in 1972 (Sciara, 1975).

In 1967 in the United States, there were six million children in fatherless homes (Herzog and Sudia, 1973). Oppel and Royston (1971) noted that of 86 mothers, only 24 fathers were there six to eight years later, in contrast to marriages of 86 mothers over age 18 in which the father of the baby was present in 50 percent of cases six to eight years later.

What does the presence of the father contribute? The data are incomplete but expanding rapidly. When the father is involved with the infant at birth or within the first few days, it leads him to have what Greenberg and Morris (1974) have termed "engrossment." Lind (1973) compared fathers who had undressed their babies twice in the first five days of the baby's life with a group of fathers who did not have that experience. Those who had changed their baby showed a significant increase in the amount of time spent with the baby in the first three months.

Paternal attachment can be enhanced by provision of a birth environment that diminishes the father's inhibitions about being involved in the birth process along with the mother. The father's participation in the birth and his attitude toward it constituted the most significant variable in predicting father attachment (Peterson et al, 1979).

Leiderman and Seashore (1975) suggested that separation in the newborn period has a nonspecific stress effect on the family that creates disequilibrium in the nuclear family structure. In studies of parents of prematures, Blake et al (1975) observed an emotional crisis in the mother which was not fully resolved until the parents began caring for the baby at home. The mothers who received sympathy and support from the baby's father appeared to have the least difficulty.

Yogman (1977) filmed infants in the first few months having different dyadic interactions with father and mother. In both cases they were mutually regulated; the partners built to a peak of attentional involvement and then decreased in an orderly cyclic manner. He postulated that father plays a unique, important, and direct role with the infant, which starts at birth and complements the mother's involvement.

Goldstein and Peck (1972), studying children age eight to 15 years in a low socioeconomic and emotionally disturbed group, found that father's presence increased the stability of the maternal childbearing activities. In the lower class black family, he was crucial to psychological differentiation, in making for a more predictable maternal cognitive effect, and in development of impulse controls (see also Sugar, 1967).

Parental loss was noted by Tandon and Tandon (1978) in 46 percent of delinquent boys versus 14 percent in a group of matched psychiatric control cases. Gregory (1965) suggested from an anterospective study that the identification model provided and the control normally exercised by the parent of the same sex are more crucial in preventing delinquency among children than is any aspect of the relation with the parent of the opposite sex.

RISK TO INFANTS

Broussard and Hartner (1970, 1971) observed that maternal perception of an infant is fluid and there is a need to emphasize support systems for the mother postpartally. The usual system of postpartal and pediatric care does not provide professional support for the mother for about six weeks postpartum. This is especially deficient when the infant is in the premature nursery, and even more so if the mother has no personal physician as is the case in clinic populations.

With the increased likelihood of a premature birth and a prolonged new-born nursery stay for the infant, the adolescent mother suffers a degree of libidinal or neonatal deprivation. Commonly, this is not decreased much when the infant comes home since the mothering is often divided with her mother or aunt, etc., which further interferes in the mother-infant bonding (Sugar, 1976).

Lewis et al (1974) described a syndrome of postpartum developmental distress in infants whose mothers had personality or emotional disorders. This was more likely to occur when an unmarried mother kept her baby, or when the premature infant was hospitalized and the mother was at home (that is, mother and infant separated). Premature infants may have a greater number of repeat hospitalizations in infancy if the father is absent, mother had no prenatal care, mother is on welfare, and there are other children in the home (Glass et al, 1971). These certainly apply to the situation with the adolescent mother who frequently has a premature offspring and who usually divides the mothering of her infant with the maternal grandmother. Illnesses of a serious type, such as those requiring hospital admission, were found in a group of abused children with much higher frequency than in the control group (Lynch, 1975).

By administering the Brazelton Neonatal Assessment Scale to infants of adolescent mothers and older mothers, Thompson et al (1979) found that the infants of the adolescent mothers were significantly less capable of responding to social stimuli, less alert, and less able to control motor behavior and perform integrated motor activities than the infants of older mothers.

Patker and associates (1961) noted that the infant death rate due to respiratory infections and accidents was more than twice as high among infants born out of wedlock than in those of married mothers. The mortality rate for infants of young mothers is very high (National Center for Health Statistics, 1971) and this is increased when they are born out of wedlock. Infants of low socioeconomic status are at high risk even if not premature or small-for-date (Knobloch and Pasamanick, 1966; Pasamanick and Knobloch, 1966). The nutritional status of the infants of adolescent mothers is deficient and causes a lag in their growth (Osofsky et al, 1973; Lloyd-Still et al, 1974).

There is increased risk for infants of adolescent mothers for becoming battered children and for failure to thrive (Helfer and Kempe, 1968; Klein and

Stern, 1971; Lynch and Roberts, 1977). Kempe and Helfer (1972) estimated that 15 percent of illness before age five is really child abuse. Adolescent mothers' children, from six to eight years, were compared with those of adult mothers and were observed to be more outgoing, dependent, and distractible. They had more behavior problems, and were more likely to be underweight and undersized (Oppel and Royston, 1971). Mothers under 17 years of age are less intensely involved with their children and have less desire to control them or keep them closely attached (Oppel and Royston, 1971; Lloyd-Still et al, 1974).

Lynch and Roberts (1977) described five factors predicting child abuse related to signs of bonding failure which they felt could be discerned in the maternity hospital immediately postpartally. These factors are the mother's age being less than 21 years at the birth of her first child, evidence of emotional disturbance in the mother, referral of the family to the hospital social worker, the baby's admission to a special care unit, and recorded concern over the mother's ability to care for the child by members of the hospital staff. In 50 percent of the cases of child abuse or neglect, the mother's age was below 20 years, versus 16 percent in a control group.

Sills and associates (1977) described a group of nonaccidental injuries in which 18 percent of the infants were premature; there was a two-to-one ratio of male to female infants and the risk to the infants increased in their second year. The average age of the mothers in this group at the birth of the first child was 19. Sixty percent of the mothers were married and one fifth of the mothers had expressed feelings of rejection of the child. It had been noted that the infant who is perhaps at greater risk for child abuse is the one who has some congenital anomaly or disturbing behavior which in some way does not invite the mother to care for it. However, none of these infants had these particular liabilities. Lenoski (1974) found a 30 percent rate of abused children among those delivered by Caesarean section compared with 3.2 percent rate for those born by vaginal delivery.

Ryan and associates (1977) showed that in 42 percent of cases the abusive guardian was identified as at high risk since it was a single parenting situation. The abuse ratio was greater for male than female children and it was most often the first child who was selected in 48 percent of cases.

Smith (1974) noted that among a series of 134 battered children, 51 percent were male, and of all the children 24 percent were premature infants. The pregnancies had been unplanned and the child was not wanted. There had been a difficult neonatal period and the child may have been handicapped, retarded, or difficult in some way since birth.

Martin (1972) observed that 33 percent of the abused children whom he studied were retarded and 43 percent had neurologic abnormalities on follow-up. He felt that the retardation was not entirely due to central nervous system damage, but was more likely due to environmental deprivation. Thus, the premature or handicapped infant is at further risk with an adolescent mother, due to the longer hospital stay with a differential in the bonding between the child and mother as well as being more subject to abuse.

Sheep illustrate the concept of a time-limited sensitive bonding period postpartally. When ewes and lambs separate during the first 30 to 45 minutes after delivery, 40 to 50 percent of the mothers fail to develop a specific attachment to the infant. If separated after two days of care for an equal period of time, the mother immediately resumes previous caretaking when reunited (Hersher et al, 1963). The infant who remains in the intensive care unit because of low birth weight or perinatal illness has an increased likelihood of difficulties due to the maternal and paternal sensitive periods not being taken advantage of to facilitate bonding and involvement with the mother and father.

Lézine et al (1975) commented on the importance of the fourth day of life for the evolution of mother-infant relationships. They found that mothers provoked more breaks in bottle-feeding on the fourth day, especially primiparous mothers of girls. The mothers felt much more able to take care of their infants after the fourth day.

From a group of 349 premature infants and a matched control group of 186 full-term infants who were observed for the onset of developmental milestones, it was found that there was a statistical difference in the onset of sitting, crawling, walking, and teething between the premature and the control infants. Sitting and walking were delayed in relation to length of separation from the mother while the teething delay was related to birth weight. Crawling delay was related to birth weight and length of separation. There was no statistical difference in the onset of stranger and separation anxiety, but there was a lag in both weight groups (premature and full-term) of about a month, in that their onset was at nine months (Sugar, 1977).

Wiener (1968) indicated risk of lower intelligence for low birth-weight babies. These findings, however, were based on studies in infants born before the modern advances in neonatology; this allows for some skepticism about the present application of those findings. Lobl and associates (1971) found that the IQ scores and the birth weight increased for black and white children proportionally to the mother's age at delivery.

Baldwin (1976), following a group of children of adolescent mothers, noted that among these children at age four, 11 percent had an IQ of 70 or less compared with only 2.6 percent of the general population; only five percent had an IQ greater than 110 compared with 25 percent of the general population (Record et al, 1969; Illsley, 1967). Werner and coworkers (1971) found that the best predictor of the children's IQ at ages two and ten years was the quality of the mother's care. From the collaborative study of 1959 to 1962, Broman and associates (1975) observed that aside from neurologic metabolic, or congenital anomalies, or other organic factors in the youngsters, the best predictors of IQ at age four years were the mother's education and socioeconomic status (SES). A lower IQ was significantly associated with the mother being under 20 and having a short pregnancy-free interval. Neligan and associates (1974) found that social factors in the family are the most significant in relation to premature infants' intelligence and that these had a greater effect on the IQ at age five years than the birth weight and outweighed perinatal factors as well. The two particular items contributing to this are the quality of the mother's care for the child at age three years and the number of live children born before the premature infant.

Douglas (1975) observed the long-term effects of early childhood hospital admission of youngsters born during the first week of March 1946 in Great Britain who were followed every two years for the next 26 years. One hospital admission of more than one week's duration or repeated admissions before the age of five years, in particular between age six months and four years, were associated with an increased risk of behavior disturbance and poor reading in adolescence. The children who had these early hospitalizations were more troublesome out of classroom, more likely to be delinquent, and more likely to show unstable job patterns than those not hospitalized in the first five years.

Lewis et al (1979) noted that perinatal difficulties and psychiatric impairment were significantly more prevalent in medical histories of incarcerated delinquents. Especially violent children had more perinatal difficulties, accidents, injuries, and ward admissions than did their less violent incarcerated peers.

Forssman and Thuwe (1966) followed 120 children born between 1939 and 1942, whose mothers had made application for abortion but had been refused. These youngsters were followed up to age 21 years along with a control group. Of the unwanted children, 60 percent had an insecure childhood. There were many complaints at home; the child had to be removed from home, put in foster care, or into a residential home. In some cases there had been parental divorce or death or the youngster had been born out of wedlock and never legitimized. The youngsters who were unwanted had significantly more psychiatric consultation, delinquency and crime, public assistance, and a lower level of higher education compared with those who had been wanted (that is, the control group youngsters).

Usually, infants see the pediatrician or family doctor for a routine check with their mothers. The infants of the adolescent mothers whom I saw for over seven years were frequently brought for their routine clinic visits by the maternal grandmother, an aunt, or a friend. Some of the mothers were never seen because they were in school, working, or had deserted the child (Sugar, 1979).

In studying the multiparous mothers, many were found to be exhibiting the same kind of absent maturity, irresponsibility, and lack of awareness of infant needs as the primiparous adolescent mothers. Quite a number of them were in their 20s and had demonstrated their parturient ability since their mid-teens, but were still functioning at the same earlier level.

The following cases are representative of some of the individual variations in a random sampling of mothers and their infants in a pediatric clinic population. Some of the problems mentioned are reflected. It should be noted that these data were not derived from an extensive or intensive interviewing or research approach to the mothers since in this study the infants were the focal point.

CASE REPORTS

Ms. A.

Unmarried Ms. A at age 15 delivered a female child, at age 16 delivered a female child, at age 23 delivered a male child, and at age 27 was pregnant with fourth child and seeking welfare.

At age 22 she developed hypertension, which fluctuated according to her diet and weight; she also used illicit drugs and alcohol. At ages 24 and 26, she was hospitalized for a schizophrenic reaction after which she gave away her two youngest children to relatives. During pregnancy at age 27, she was in remission from the schizophrenic reaction while taking antipsychotic drugs, but she had psychotic symptoms. She had a seventh-grade education and tested as a borderline retardate. Now she wanted to regain custody of the two children.

Ms. B.

An unwed 18-year-old adolescent mother deserted her first-born, a girl, one week postpartally and returned five months later to assist the grandmother in raising the child. She noted at the six month's examination that the baby was quiet and wondered if she should be concerned. At age eight months, the infant had not gained weight for two months. At nine months, "the baby would not go to anyone but the grandparents" and showed stranger anxiety reactions to the mother. At ten months the infant had a 6 oz weight loss recorded since the last visit. A diagnosis of a failure-to-thrive infant was made.

Ms. C.

At age 3.5 months her male infant was brought to the clinic by the unwed mother's 15-year-old age-mate girlfriend who quoted the mother as "[stopping] him from thumbsucking 'cause grandmother said to." At 15 months, he was brought by his 16-year-old maternal aunt who said he was being punched by the mother for gritting his teeth. At 24 months he was diagnosed as asthmatic, for which he had had three hospital trips in the previous five months. This youngster seemed on the road to becoming a battered child.

Ms. D.

This 13-year-old mother, who had returned to school postpartally, complained that her female infant who was being raised by the maternal grandmother did not recognize the mother at six months and cried when the mother took her. The baby had bronchiolitis at six months, impetigo at 21 months, and pneumonia at 24 months.

Ms. E.

At age 18, this married mother delivered a full-term female infant. Five weeks later when she returned to school, the care of the infant was divided between the mother and a two-year-younger maternal aunt. This continued for some three months until the family relocated in another city when the mother began to work full time and the infant was placed in an all-day nursery. The infant was described as being very quiet and manifesting rumination until 15 months. The mother was not able to clearly recall the child's developmental milestones.

When the child was age three, a male sibling was born. The mother stayed home for five weeks and then took a vacation trip with the father. On her return, the older child was noted to be angry and withdrawn but the mother returned to full-time work immediately. The care of the younger child was continued by others while the older child attended an all-day nursery. At age four it was noted that the girl rarely spoke, which was brought to the mother's attention by the nursery school personnel. Instead of making her needs known verbally, she had them passed on through a girl cousin of about the same age who was the spokesman. Thus, the little girl had found herself a mother surrogate who took care of her needs. She was diagnosed as having marked separation anxiety with severe restriction in social functioning with peers and other adults beyond her parents and cousin.

Cases C and D support the relationship of a higher risk for illness in premature infants of adolescent mothers without a father and an uninvolved mother. Cases A, B, D, and E point to problems in mother infant bonding (see Chapters 4, 5, and 8, this volume).

Thus, we see the strange and frightening world of the unwed adolescent mother and her child. She cannot joyfully anticipate the birth of her child. She is woefully unprepared to plan and provide for it. She has neither the knowledge nor the emotional maturity to mother it wisely. Beset by many problems, she often becomes ambivalent to her child and later develops a total lack of commitment to the infant. This is reflected by the complications in pregnancy, labor, and delivery, and by the complications that ensue physically, nutritionally, and congenitally, all of which affect the infant's development, its bonding with the mother and the father, and its later development emotionally. She appears unprepared for marriage or motherhood and more in need of a mother or mother-surrogate for herself.

CONCLUSIONS

The research data presented in this chapter on infants of adolescents emphasize their being at risk. Such children have a mother who has not completed her own optimal physical, cognitive, and emotional development and is in need of much support and counselling to avoid complications in pregnancy, labor, bonding, and caring for the infant.

Without intervention, these infants face high rates for neonatal mortality, prematurity, and neonatal morbidity with attendant separation from their mother. Bonding and developmental difficulties are implicated in the high probability they face for failure to thrive, abuse, neglect, nutritional and intellectual difficulties, as well as physical illness. The data suggest the absence of normal matresence in the adolescent girl.

Programs for counselling and teaching the mother how to mother appropriately, stimulate, accept, and bond with her infant offer significant possibilities for prevention. By these interventions, complications or interferences in the infants' development may hopefully be avoided or decreased.

REFERENCES

Anastasiow, N. J., Everett, M., O'Shaughnessy, T. E., Eggleston, P. J. and Eklund, S. J. 1978. Improving teenage attitudes toward children, child handicaps and hospital settings. *Am. J. Orthopsychiatry* 48:663–672.

Baldwin, W. H. 1976. Adolescent pregnancy and childbearing—growing concern for Americans. *Popul. Bull.* 31(2).

Beric, B., Bregun, N. and Bujas, M. 1978. Obstetric aspects of adolescent pregnancy and delivery. *Int. J. Gynaecol. Obstet.* 15:491–493.

Blake, A., Stewart, A. and Turcan, D. 1975. Parents of babies of very low birth weight: long term follow-up. In *Parent-Infant Interaction.* Ciba Foundation Symposium #33. Amsterdam, North Holland: Elsevier-Excerpta Medica.

Broman, S., Nicholls, P. and Kennedy, W. 1975. *Preschool I.Q.* Hillsdale, New Jersey: Earlbaum Associates.

Brown, J. V. and Bakeman, R. 1977. *Antecedents of Emotional Involvement in Mothers of Premature and Fullterm Infants.* Presented at the Society for Research in Child Development meeting. New Orleans, March 1977.

Broussard, E. R. and Hartner, M. S. S. 1970. Maternal perception of the neonate as related to development. *Child Psych. Hum. Dev.* 1:16–25.

Broussard, E. R. and Hartner, M. S. S. 1971. Further considerations regarding maternal perception of the first-born. In J. Hellmuth (Ed.): *Exceptional Infant. Vol. II. Studies in Abnormalities.* New York: Brunner/Mazel.

Collingwood, J. and Alberman, E. 1979. Separation at birth and the mother-child relationship. *Dev. Med. Child Neurol.* 21:608–618.

Cutright, P. 1972. The teenage sexual revolution and the myth of an abstinent past. *Fam. Plann. Perspect.* 4:24–31.

Douglas, J. W. B. 1975. Early hospital admissions and later disturbances of behaviour and learning. *Dev. Med. Child Neurol.* 17:456–480.

Erickson, J. D. 1978. Down's syndrome, paternal age, maternal age and birth order. *Ann. Hum. Genet.* 41:289–298.

Erkan, K. A., Rimer, B. A. and Stine, O. C. 1971. Juvenile pregnancy: role of physiologic maturity. *Maryland State Med. J.* 20:50–52.

Eskin, B. 1977. When do nocturnal emissions begin in adolescence? *Med. Trib.*

Forssman, H. and Thuwe, I. 1966. One hundred and twenty children born after application for therapeutic abortion refused. *Acta Psychiat. Scand.* 42: 71–78.

Glass, L., Kolko, N. and Evans, H. 1971. Factors influencing predispositions to serious illness in low birth weight infants. *Pediatrics* 48:368–371.

Goldstein, H. S. and Peck, R. 1972. Maternal differentiation, father absence and cognitive differentiation in children. *Arch. Gen. Psychiatry* 29:370–373.

Greenberg, M. and Morris, N. 1974. Engrossment: the newborn's impact upon the father. *Am. J. Orthopsychiatry* 44:520–531.

Gregory, I. 1965. Anterospective data following childhood loss of a parent. *Arch. Gen. Psychiatry* 13:99–107.

Hales, D. J., Kennell, J., Klaus, M., Mata, L., Sosa, R. and Urrutia, J. 1975. The effect of early skin to skin contact on maternal behavior at twelve hours. *Pediatr. Res.* 9:259.

Hales, D. J., Lozoff, B., Sosa, R. and Kennell, J. H. 1977. Defining the limits of the maternal sensitive period. *Dev. Med. Child Neurol.* 19:454–461.

Hanson, J. W., Jones, K. L. and Smith, D. W. 1976. Fetal alcohol syndrome. *J.A.M.A.* 235:1458–60.

Helfer, R. E. and Kempe, C. H. 1968. *The Battered Child.* Chicago: University of Chicago Press.

Hersher, L., Richmond, J. and Moore, A. 1963. Modifiability of the critical period for the development of maternal behavior in sheep and goats. *Int. J. Comp. Ethol.* 20:311–320.

Herzog, E. and Sudia, C. E. 1973. Children in fatherless families. In B. M. Caldwell and H. A. Ricciuti (Eds.): *Review of Child Development Research.* Chicago: University of Chicago Press, Vol. 3, pp. 141–232.

Illsley, R. 1967. Family growth and its effect on the relationship between obstetric factors and child functioning. In P. Roberts and A. S. Parker (Eds.): *Social and Genetic Influences on Life and Death.* London: Oliver and Boyd.

Jekel, J. F., Harrison, J. T., Bancroft, D. R. E., Tyler, N. C. and Klerman, L. V. 1975. A comparison of the subsequent health of index and subsequent babies born to school age mothers. *Am. J. Publ. Health* 65:370–374.

Jones, K. L. and Smith, D. W. 1973. Recognition of the fetal alcohol syndrome in early infancy. *Lancet* 2:999–1001.

Jones, K. L. and Smith, D. W. 1975. The fetal alcohol syndrome. *Teratology* 12: 1–10.

Katz, I. B., Brenner, B. N. and Sarzin, B. 1977. Pregnancy in the unwed white South African. *South African Med. J.* 52:79–81.

Kempe, C. H. and Helfer, R. E. 1972. *Helping the Battered Child and His Family*. 2nd ed. Philadelphia: J. B. Lippincott.

Kennell, J. H., Jerauld, R., Wolfe, H., Chesler, D., Kreger, N. C., McAlpine, W., Steffa, M. and Klaus, M. H. 1974. Maternal behavior one year after early and extended post-partum contact. *Dev. Med. Child. Neurol.* 16:172–179.

Kihss, P. 1977. *New York Times*. September 29, p. 39.

Klein, M. and Stern, L. 1971. Low birth weight and the battered child syndrome. *Am. J. Dis. Child.* 122:15–18.

Knobloch, H. and Pasamanick, B. 1966. Prospective studies on the epidemiology of reproductive casualty, methods, findings and some implications. *Merrill-Palmer Q.* 12:27–43.

Leiderman, P. H. and Seashore, M. J. 1975. Mother-infant neonatal separation: some delayed consequences. In *Parent-Infant Interaction*. Ciba Foundation Symposium #33. Amsterdam, North Holland: Elsevier-Excerpta Medica.

Lenoski, E. F. 1974. Unpublished manuscript quoted by Parke R. D. and Collimer, C. W. 1975. Child abuse: an inter-disciplinary analysis. In E. M. Hetherington (Ed.): *Review of Child Development Research*, Vol. 5. Chicago: University of Chicago Press, pp. 509–590.

Lewis, D. O., Shanok, S. S. and Balla, D. A. 1979. Perinatal difficulties, head and face trauma and child abuse in medical histories of seriously delinquent children. *Am. J. Psychiatry* 136:419–429.

Lewis, P. J. E., McKinnon, P., Simms, C. W. R. and Ironside, W. 1974. The Karitane project: psychological ill-health, infant distress and the post-partum period. *N.Z. Med. J.* 79:1005–1009.

Lézine, I., Robin, M. and Cortial, C. 1975. Observations sur le couple mère-enfant au cours des premières experiences alimentaires. *Psychiatr. Enfant* 18:75–146.

Lind, J. 1973. Quoted by Kennell J. 1975. In *Parent-Infant Interaction*. Ciba Foundation Symposium #33. Amsterdam, North Holland: Elsevier-Excerpta Medica, p. 65.

Lloyd-Still, J. D., Hurwitz, E., Wolff, P. H. and Shwachman, H. 1974. Intellectual development after severe malnutrition in infancy. *Pediatrics* 54:306–311.

Lobl, M., Welcher, D. W. and Mellits, E. D. 1971. Maternal age and intellectual functioning of offspring. *Johns Hopkins Med. J.* 128:347–361.

Lowe, C. R. 1959. Effects of mothers' smoking habits on birth weight of their children. *Br. Med. J.* 2:673–676.

Lynch, M. A. 1975. Ill-health and child abuse. *Lancet* 2:317–319.

Lynch, M. A. and Roberts, J. 1977. Predicting child abuse: signs of bonding failure in the maternity hospital. *Br. Med. J.* 1:624–626.

Martin, H. 1972. The child and his development. In C. H. Kempe and R. E. Helfer (Eds.): *Helping the Battered Child and His Family*. Philadelphia: J. B. Lippincott.

Mikkelson, M. 1967. Down's syndrome at young maternal age: cytogenetical and genealogical study of 82 families. *Ann. Hum. Genet.* 31:59–69.

National Center for Health Statistics. 1981. Infant Mortality Rates by Legitimacy Status: United States 1964–1966. *Monthly Vital Statistics Rep.* 20:5.

National Institute on Alcohol Abuse and Alcoholism. 1977. *Critical Review of the Fetal Alcohol Syndrome.* Rockville, Maryland: Alcohol, Drug Abuse, and Mental Health Administration.

Neligan, G., Prudham, D. and Steiner, H. 1974. *Formative Years: Birth, Family and Development in Newcastle upon Tyne.* Oxford: Oxford University Press.

Oppel, W. C. and Royston, A. B. 1971. Teen-age births: some social, psychological and physical sequelae. *Am. J. Publ. Health* 61:751–756.

Osofsky, H. J., Osofsky, J. D., Kendall, N. and Rajan, R. 1973. Adolescents as mothers: an interdisciplinary approach to a complex problem. *J. Youth Adol.* 2:233–249.

Pakter, J., Ranes, H., Jacobziner, H. and Greensteen, F. 1961. Out of wedlock births in New York City. II. Medical aspects. *Am. J. Publ. Health* 51: 846–865.

Pasamanick, B. and Knobloch, H. 1966. Retrospective studies on the epidemiology of reproductive casualty: old and new. *Merrill-Palmer Q.* 12:7–26.

Peterson, G. H., Mehl, L. E. and Leiderman, P. H. 1979. The role of some birth-related variables in father attachment. *Am. J. Orthopsychiatry* 49(2):330–338.

Raphael, D. 1973. *The Tender Gift.* New Jersey: Prentice Hall.

Record, G., McKeowon, T. and Edwards, J. H. 1969. The relation of measured intelligence to birth order and maternal age. *Ann. Hum. Genet.* 33:51–69.

Ringler, N. M., Kennell, H., Jarvella, R., Navojosky, B. J. and Klaus, M. H. 1975. Mother-to-child speech at 2 years—effects of early postnatal contact. *J. Pediatr.* 86:141–144.

Ringler, N., Trause, M., Klaus, M., and Kennell, J. 1978. The effects of extra postpartum contact and maternal speech patterns on children's IQs, speech, and language comprehension at five. *Child Dev.* 49:862–865.

Ryan, M. G., Davis, A. A. and Oates, R. K. 1977. One hundred and eighty-seven cases of child abuse and neglect. *Med. J. Aust.* 2:623–628.

Ruppersberg, A. 1973. Maternal deaths among Ohio teenagers—a 16 year study. *Ohio State Med. J.* 69:692–694.

Sciara, F. J. 1975. Effects of father absence on the educational achievement of urban black children. *Child Study J.* 5:45–55.

Sills, J. A., Thoman, L. H. and Rosenbloom, L. 1977. Non-accidental injury: a two year study in central Liverpool. *Dev. Med. Child Neurol.* 19:26–33.

Simpson, W. J. A. 1957. Preliminary report on cigarette smoking and the incidence of prematurity. *Am. J. Obstet. Gynecol.* 73:808–815.

Smith, P. B., Mumford, D. M., Goldfarb, J. L. and Kaufman, R. H. 1975. Selected aspects of adolescent post partum behavior. *J. Reproduct. Med.* 14:159–165.

Smith, S. M. 1974. One hundred and thirty-four battered children; a medical and psychological study. *Br. Med. J.* 3:666–670.

Sturt, R. J. and Sturt, A. B. 1974. Natality, fertility and marriage status in Sepik River population of New Guinea. *Trop. Geogr. Med.* 26:399–413.

Sugar, M. 1967. Group therapy for pubescent boys with absent fathers. *J. Am. Acad. Child Psychiatry* 6:478–498.

Sugar, M. 1976. At risk factors for the adolescent mother and her infant. *J. Youth Adol.* 5:251–270.

Sugar, M. 1977. Some milestones in premature infants at six to twenty-four months. *Child Psych. Hum. Dev.* 8:67–80.

Sugar, M. 1979. Developmental Aspects of Adolescent Motherhood. In M. Sugar (Ed.): *Female Adolescent Development.* New York: Brunner/Mazel.

Tandon, A. K. and Tandon, R. K. 1978. Parental deprivation and delinquency. *Indian Pediatr.* 15:33–38.

Thoman, E. B. 1975. How a rejecting baby affects mother-infant synchrony. In *Parent-Infant Interaction.* Ciba Foundation Symposium #33. Amsterdam, North Holland: Elsevier-Excerpta Medica.

Thompson, R. J., Cappleman, M. W. and Zeitschel, K. A. 1979. Neonatal behavior of infants of adolescent mothers. *Dev. Med. Child Neurol.* 21:474–482.

Waters, J. 1969. Pregnancy in young adolescents. *South Med. J.* 62:655–658.

Werner, E., Bierman, J. and French, P. 1971. *The Children of Kauai.* Honolulu: University Press of Hawaii.

Wiener, G. 1968. Scholastic achievement at age 12–13 of prematurely born infants. *J. Special Ed.* 2:237–250.

Yogman, N. W. 1977. *The Goals and Structure of Face-to-Face Interaction between Infants and Fathers.* Presented at the Society for Research in Child Development Meeting. New Orleans, March 1977.

Zelnick, M. and Kantner, J. F. 1974. The resolution of teenage first pregnancies. *Fam. Plann. Perspect.* 6:74–80.

Zelnick, M. and Kantner, J. F. 1978. First pregnancies to women aged 15–19: 1976 and 1971. *Fam. Plann. Perspect.* 10:11–19.

8

Object Ties and Interaction of the Infant and Adolescent Mother

JO ANN B. FINEMAN
AND MARGUERITE A. SMITH

Lady Capulet. Well, think of marriage now. Younger than you here in Vernoa, ladies of esteem, are made already mothers. By my count, I was your mother much upon these years that you are now a maid.

Romeo and Juliet. Act I, Scene iii
William Shakespeare

The familiar wrangle between Lady Capulet and the Nurse, one exhorting Juliet to marry and bear children, the other remembering her infancy and nursing days, brings to a sharp focus the dilemma of the adolescent child mothers we have seen in our clinical services over the past several years. The graceful language of Shakespeare is not often duplicated in the pained and bitter conflicts between the adolescent mother and her own mother, as each struggles to contend with the merging and antagonistic developmental phases which are forced upon them with the coming of the child-mother's baby.

If we assume, as Lichtenberg (1975) does, that "the foundation for the psychic dimension of infantile life is formed from the basic 'fit' between mother and infant," and that this fit depends on the ongoing reciprocal attunement of the mother to the infant's sensorimotor and affect experiences and messages, we must then look for the observable interactions which allow us to become aware of the congruence or dissonance of this fit.

Lichtenberg (1975) further stated, referring to Weil (1972) and others, that these early interactions foreshadow the outlines of later ego-id functions and, by inference, defenses and sublimations, as well as object-relatedness.

119

Object relations have come to indicate a broad spectrum of behaviors, intra-psychic images, and theoretical assumptions. For the purposes of this chapter, we will concentrate on the quality of loving and trust building in the early rela-tionship between the infant of the adolescent mother and her mothering of this infant, as we have observed these dyads and have speculated about the outcomes in our clinical material and observations. Soothing and comforting experiences between this dyad must be dominant, if later self-representations are to be sup-portive of benign and appropriate self-love, and the containment and modifica-tion of aggressive fantasies and actions of the later toddler and child. Following Edgecumbe and Bergner (1972), we would understand our material in the light of the statement that "what is cathected at this early stage is the representative of an experiential state, not a representation of the self." Such a concept is vividly dramatic when viewed in the context of our clinical observations of adolescent mothers and their infants.

There is a cautionary inference to be made here, lest we be seen as starkly pessimistic or negative in our formulations of these mothers and infants. We can-not rule out a dyadic fit which promotes the early soothing and tension-reducing experience in the infant, but our clinical evidence, gathered over a period of seven years, indicates that such a fit is a rarity in our population of inner-city adolescent mothers. The confluence of adolescence and motherhood seems to exacerbate contending inner forces in the girl-mother, as we suggest in our later discussion.

DATA BASE

In our clinical services for "high risk" babies and their mothers, we have followed a total of 167 families. We wish to highlight the characteristics of the teenage mothers and provide some data about the total population in order to place these findings in context.

Our unit is located in inner-city Boston and serves a population that is virtually 100 percent "at risk." Recent figures from the Boston City Hospital's Neonatology Department report that from 75 to 80 percent of babies born there have some "less than favorable" characteristic at birth, and that from 30 to 35 percent of babies have some obvious diagnosable birth defect or anomaly of a permanent nature. This is in contrast to figures of well below 1 percent per year in a nearby largely private suburban hospitals.

The incidence of adolescent pregnancy in this general area cannot be specifically stated. But current data from one of the large inner-city high schools indicates that in the academic year 1978–1979, the verified pregnancy rate of young women in this high school was 18.78 percent. This figure of almost 19 percent approaches the highest reported in any population group studied in the

United States according to any presently available statistics. In addition, this is an area in which the majority of families are at poverty level or live in marginal socioeconomic conditions.

Furthermore, in a large part of this inner city, the infant mortality rate is the highest of any area in the state and has been found to be 29 deaths per 1,000 live births, compared with the national figure 15 per 1,000. Expectedly, other statistics indicating serious and early maladaptation between infant and caretaker can be seen to concentrate on this at risk population. Roughly 50 percent of reported cases derived at least part of their income from general relief or Aid to Families of Dependent Children.

Since mothers and babies are referred to us as "at risk" dyads across a spectrum that ranges from "baby has problem at birth" to "mother's situation is high risk factor," we approached our analysis from several angles: for example, age of mother at birth of baby, condition of baby at birth, severity of baby's problem, reason for referral, age of baby at referral, stability of mother's home situation. Finally, each family was rated on a scale from 1 to 5 on the basis of participation in the program—that is, *not* in terms of the quality of mothering or state of the infant, but solely on such concrete items as "keeps appointment, is home for scheduled home visits, keeps scheduled clinic appointments, stays with program for duration of need or until referral to further appropriate program," etc. This caused some difficulty for staff, because it does not correlate with the subjective judgment of the *quality* of mothering, so that some of our most troublesome families would turn out to be rated 1 (highest). The converse is not true. Mothers rated 4 or 5 did not include any whose mothering was otherwise seen as "good" or "adequate" by staff. The rating reflects the availability of the family to the treatment team, without a judgment of success of response to treatment.

We were particularly interested in exploring the group of teenage mothers, which totalled 52, ranging in age from 14 to 19 at the time of the baby's birth. Further examination of this group led us almost immediately to a further age classification. Since "very young mother" was established with our referring sources as an adequate reason for an at risk referral, this introduced a bias in our younger-age samples that became evident as we explored "reason for referral." Very young mother was the sole reason for referral in the 14- to 17-year-old group, but with the 18- to 19-year-old girls there was a shift to a combination of age of mother plus an additional at risk factor. It became evident that in general the 14- to 17-year-old mother was psychologically in a very different position from the 18- to 20-year-old mother. First (at least in our group), the 14 to 17 year olds were still part of their primary family, living at home, with little or no contact or continuing affiliation with the father of the baby. None had finished high school at the time of pregnancy and birth of the baby. Some specifically used the pregnancy as a reason for leaving school, even when other arrangements were offered to them.

Further credibility is given to the developmental differentiation between middle and later adolescent mothers by another sample. In a subsequent study, we surveyed a group of 34 high school girls—aged approximately 14 to 17 years—who delivered babies during the academic year 1978-1979. Of this group, over 75 percent stayed in the parental (often only maternal) home and devised a system of shared child care with their own mothers or a close female relative. Of these 34 girls, only five decided to move away from home and attempt to establish themselves in an independent living situation apart from their families of origin.

In contrast, most of the 18- to 19-year-old girls had moved away from the family home or used the pregnancy as a reason for this move, had or continued to have an affiliation with the father of the baby, had either finished high school or been involved in some self-supporting work that took them out of the home, even if they continued technically to live there. That is to say, either from their own volition or because of pressures from the family of origin, these girls were already breaking away from their parental figures.

One should note also the reflection of the societal evaluation of the 18 to 20 years olds versus the 14 to 17 year olds in that for the older group, age alone was insufficient reason for referral as a high risk mother. One feature that characterized the very young mother group was both surprising and interesting to us: the babies in the group were healthier than those in the other referral groups, although nine babies were premature—a 36 percent rate of prematurity! Only three babies had birth defects that would have occasioned a referral to us regardless of the mother's age. And, oddly enough, these were three unusual and unusually serious problems: a triple amputee, a hemophiliac baby, and a baby described as a "prune belly." One needs to remember the built-in skew in this group when we state these babies were the healthiest of the age groups in our sample, that is, the fact that *age alone* could be the reason for referral. It should be stressed, however, that while we surely did not have every pregnant girl under 17 years in the area referred to us, we would have had every "problem baby" born at Boston City Hospital to this age group referred to us. In other words, babies of 14 to 17 year olds *not* referred would have been healthy babies whose family support systems for the young mother were seen as adequate, for whom our services were not needed.

Of particular importance for the focus of this chapter is the fact that in this group of very young mothers, almost all the babies started out as healthy with all indications of developing normally and so deserve our best efforts of preventive intervention.

The most discouraging item about this group was that of all the high risk groups, it provided the most difficulty and was the poorest in ratings of "availability of the family to the treatment team." In terms of moderate to severe problems of the baby, all other groups showed about an even split in highly rated versus poorly rated families, but in this group of young mothers with healthy babies the distribution was four to one against "accessibility to the family." Specifically, of the 25 mother/infant dyads in this group, only four remained in good contact with the program, and 16 were essentially lost to follow-up.

Unfortunately, we know more than we would like to know about what happens to that group of mothers and babies with whom we lost contact altogether. Many of them are similar to the mothers who make up our next line of referrals to the infant program according to age—the 18 to 20 year olds, now with their second or third baby. They include those for whom the additional risk factor on the referral form frequently is "previous baby removed from her care; mother wishes to keep this baby; needs help." The sample of toddlers and preschoolers from our child psychiatry clinic can show us the impact of the mother-infant interaction on these first babies as they become two, three, and four years old.

PSYCHOPATHOLOGY IN PRESCHOOLERS WITH ADOLESCENT MOTHERS

Our preschool clinical unit accepts referrals of preschool children identified either by their day care or prekindergarten facilities, or by outreach consultative services to the neighborhood facilities. Over the past two years, from approximately 30 children whom we were able to engage in some form of evaluative procedure, we found one third had been born when their mothers were 17 years old or younger—some approaching Juliet's age of almost 14.

Their psychopathology centered around the capacity to attach and remain attached to caregiving figures and poor or incomplete modification of primitive aggression. Phrases such as "persistent maladaptive ego disturbances—either withdrawal or uncontrolled aggressive outbursts" crop up with discouraging frequency in the case summaries of these children of adolescent mothers. We found that most often we settled on the diagnosis of developmental deviation to describe the failure of consistent loving object attachment and the frequent occurrence of wildly aggressive attacks directed toward adults or peers who frustrated or tried to limit them, or *who were approaching them with nurturing and loving behavior*.

All of these children of adolescent mothers referred to our service when they were three to five years of age had failed to achieve age-appropriate internal controls over their hostile destructive impulses and actions, and were fragile in their capacity to love consistently and to accept loving approaches from their caregivers. The fact that we have used the term *caregivers* is significant; our observation from the clinical data is that more often than not the biological mother—the adolescent—loses in her struggle to be both mother and developing girl, and, through some external intervention of societal mechanisms, the baby is placed in a foster home usually before the age of two years or thereabouts. At the time of referral only four of the 30 children were in a home which included the biological mother, and two of these had been in previous foster home placement for several months.

CASE ILLUSTRATION

Terry, a prototypical child in the preschool clinical unit, had been in two foster homes by age five years. In an intensive summer program, where he was in a full day group of four children, any situation in which he had to share food or toys elicited a rage reaction. He attacked and scratched his caregivers or ran away into the surrounding vacant lots. Once he broke a glass and tried to stab himself in a self-directed destructive rage. When he finally could be held and contained, he sobbed but could not cling to the adult comforter. Terry lives in a foster home. From time to time his biological mother, who was barely 16 when he was born, visits him with the welfare worker. His mother approaches him with clear ambivalence and can only relate to him when one of the other adults takes them both to a restaurant, a nearby zoo, or amusement park. Within the triad which includes the older woman social worker, his mother can play and talk to Terry, and he has been able to hold her hand or run toward her, only to pull away when any attempt is made to reach out to him. He repeats the same behavioral evidence of failure to achieve sustained object attachment to his foster mother and to the therapists in our unit in his group milieu. He (in common with most of the children of adolescent mothers we have seen) resorts to aggressive, destructive, and impulsive behavior when involved in close contact with adults, as though the unconscious need is to ward off attachments or to protect himself against closeness which is experienced as pain-producing rather than pleasure-giving.

Since we have seen a number of adolescent mothers over the past seven years, the best exposition of the problems faced by these families can be given by the story of two contrasting girls and their families. We have attempted to study this problem by means of data regarding the individual dynamics of each case, and by an attempt to derive from the conscious and unconscious verbal and observational material some insights into the failures of adaptation and the frustration of the mother's adolescent needs that has occurred.

CONTRIBUTIONS TO ATTACHMENT DISORDERS FROM ADOLESCENT MOTHERING

From our theoretical formulations and from the clinical case studies of adolescents in treatment, we can make some predictive statements about why the 14- to 17-year age group might be expected to be a high risk group in terms of the capacity to mother. The two case vignettes presented here illustrate a point which needs strong emphasis: that intercurrent problems of maternal attachment and of the infant's developmental progress are not primarily socio-economic, but are fundamentally psychological.

The adolescent girl, in the earlier phases of the adolescent passage, has experienced a revival of longings for a reenactment of her earlier wishes for need fulfillment from her own mother, in clashing contrast to her emerging sexual arousal and the behaviors which express her sexuality. The *incidental* quality of the infant conceived in this psychic turmoil is evident if the girl's dominant wish for a repetition of her former need-satisfying experiences from her own mother are kept in mind. This emphasizes the conception of the infant in light of the earlier image of the relationship to the adolescent's mother, and not as the fulfillment of later sexual-oedipal strivings related to the unconscious wishes directed toward the adolescent's father. The girl in early adolescence creates a baby in order to identify with this infant and herself receive mothering once more. When formulated in this way, the clinical evidence that the girl-mother may be unable to forego her own needs for love and nurturance in the service of providing such experiences for her infant is soon clear. Some of the pseudo-independent rebellion and overt conflict between adolescent mother and grand-mother can be understood as a premature and fragile defense against these longings, supported by the grandmother's disappointments and failure to be able to meet her daughter's needs.

THE FAMILY MATRIX OF ATTACHMENT DISORDERS

Case 1

We first came to know the Franklin family when Diane, at 14—the mother of an 11-month-old daughter—was taken to court by her mother after a fracas in which Diane had drawn a knife on her mother and tried to stab her. Her mother had warded off the blow, and Diane had turned on her boyfriend (her baby Sally's father) in a wild and violent gesture of desperation and stabbed him. His wound was not severe, but he and the grandmother were so angered they pressed charges and requested placement for her outside the home. Since the court wisely sensed the need for psychiatric intervention, Diane was sent to us for evaluation in addition to the placement.

The Franklin family proved to be a complex and fragmented one. The gradmother was a large, tired-looking, but domineering woman who fiercely held onto her role as the principal caregiver of the three babies of her daughters, aged two years, 11 months, and seven months. Diane's older sister, now 16, had completely abdicated her role as mother after giving birth to the two year old and the seven month old, and returned to high school for the second time.

Diane, just past 14 when Sally was born, was caught in the struggle for possession of her baby but, in contradiction, could perform no caregiving without her
mother at her side to instruct her. Diane laughed and giggled when the therapist
called her "mother" and turned to grandmother for answers to inquiries regarding developmental information. In the interview, the grandmother presided,
holding the seven-month-old against her breast while Sally toddled aimlessly
about the room, looking detached and fretful.

They were poor and lived in a crowded housing project apartment. One
daughter, the eldest of the five children, had been able to leave the family and
was in college. She visited and clearly cared for her mother, but had removed
herself from the struggles of her two younger sisters. Her emancipation had been
successful, and she guarded her freedom carefully. At home were the next two
daughters, aged 16 and 14; a 12-year-old brother who was withdrawn and obese;
an eight-year-old daughter; and the grandfather. He was a cantankerous, angry
man, disabled from a stroke, who spent his time on the living room sofa, sometimes lunging at one of the girls when the arguments became fierce. The grandmother clearly ruled the home, but she had been unable to accept advice to put
her husband in a nursing home. He seemed to be another fractious and dependent child in a home where feeding and fighting anchored grandmother to each
person there; and only the oldest had escaped.

The point at which we began the evaluation seemed to be the beginning
of disintegration. Had the court intervention not taken place, we probably never
would have seen this family. The disintegration and the loss of the oldest
daughter represented a fulfillment of the wish to separate, but at the same time
mobilized guilt and regressive longings on Diane's part, and reactivated the
grandmother's need to have the children dependent and under her control.
Frank, the obese and isolated 12-year-old, had capitulated to the infantile role,
but Diane fought against it overtly, while she allowed her mother to take over
Sally's care.

Sally, the 11-month-old baby, had walked early—by nine or ten months—
but seemed to be unresponsive and had not become focused on either her
mother or grandmother for special comforting or interacting. She handled toys
awkwardly and without pleasure. Her most consistent behavior was wandering,
briefly touching or reaching for her grandmother or another adult, then just as
briefly manipulating a toy, circling her environment without settling on any one
person or thing. She could be held and, with effort from an adult, fix her gaze
onto a caregiving adult, but seemed anxious and tense when she was put in this
close contact, preferring the distance and movement.

We theorized that she represented motorically the incomplete bonding
between family members, and that in the household everyone moved together
then apart, never settling nor separating. An attempt to engage Diane and her
baby in our therapeutic program, covering several months of intense outreach

work by a staff member, proved almost fruitless. Despite home visits and the involvement of Grandmother Franklin in our baby group, both adolescent mothers decathected their infants and, possibly as a defensive position to ward off their own deep longings for a return to an infantile nurturant relationship with their own mother, yielded the mothering function to the grandmother. Diane's next older sister (who was 16) stayed in high school but psychologically abandoned her baby. Diane became more and more overtly hostile toward Grandmother Franklin and drew away from the family, turning toward a street culture which seemed to offer her a representation of the nurturance and dyadic union which she had not found within her own actuality.

Case 2

Sareta had just turned 14 when Tony was born. She is the oldest of six children, with one sister and four younger brothers. Her youngest brother was three at the time of Tony's birth. After the birth of this youngest child, the maternal grandmother had had a miscarriage, which reportedly precipitated a depression severe enough that the welfare agency allowed her to take a job specifically "prescribed" as a form of therapy.

Sareta, a shy, pudgy, sad-looking child at 14, seemed more like a ten year old than a beginning teenager. Perhaps this accounts for the fact that no one in the family realized she was pregnant until she was nearly into her sixth month, although the level of denial this requires of this large family strains credibility. Sareta herself seems to have been confused and uncertain about what was happening to her. She had little or no understanding or knowledge of sex or reproduction. She had become pregnant after her first menstrual period when she was in the sixth grade.

In spite of the fact that she seems to have been a victim of a seduction by a young man known to the family, when the pregnancy was confirmed, her parents directed their rage only against her. Her father, particularly, became furious, and struck and pushed her out of the house. When he was persuaded to let her return, he refused to speak to her for weeks on end, while he laid down very strict rules for her, kept her out of school, and required that she take over almost all of the household responsibility while her mother continued to work.

This was not a completely new situation for Sareta, since she had often been required to stay home from school to care for the younger children and for a long time had been the one who did a major share of the cooking for this family of eight.

When the mother and baby were referred to us shortly after the baby's birth, much pressure was put on the grandparents by a social worker from the neighborhood health clinic for the grandmother to leave her job to take care of her children, including Sareta. But the grandmother continued to work and

Sareta continued to have total care of the household, now adding to this already heavy burden the care of her own baby. Thus, from the beginning, this baby was placed in a position of being like one more younger brother requiring her care. As if to emphasize this, the baby's crib was kept in the grandparent's bedroom, while Sareta shared a bedroom with her younger sister and three-year-old brother.

During this period, the grandfather was almost always at home, since his main occupation as a carpenter at that time was remodeling their house. This meant that Sareta was constantly under his surveillance and subject to his outbursts of rage.

Meanwhile, there developed a good deal of open competition over the "ownership" of the baby. In spite of his continuing anger and his refusal to soften his feelings toward Sareta, the grandfather spent much time with the baby and took over much of the caretaking, even as he worked. When the grandmother returned from work, she too spent time with this baby, leaving Sareta to get dinner and care for the other children.

Visits with Sareta at home were chaotic, and attempts to understand her role and feelings about the care of this baby were difficult at best. Both grandparents seemed suspicious and resentful of our interest in Sareta and her baby, always finding some way for one or the other of them to be present for our home visits, often with several of the younger children. It was almost impossible to talk to Sareta alone, or to have any opportunity to see her with her own baby. Even under these circumstances, Sareta managed to convey how miserable she was, how she wished so much to be allowed to go to school, and also how much she resented her parents' usurpation of the baby.

The clinical team working with this troubled family had to yield to the disorganization and give up attempts for direct family therapy at this time. It seemed possible to focus on Sareta and her baby, and thus attempt a gradual integration of the family around this adolescent mother-infant dyad.

Throughout this time, the baby seemed healthy since observations of his growth and development, both at home and at the unit, showed him to be steadily at or above his age level. He was, however, from the beginning, regarded as a "serious baby" and while never seen as depressed, he was frequently described as "placid," "quiet," or "reserved," in contrast to the highly volatile emotional level of the rest of the household.

In the fall, when Tony was about nine months old, the grandmother rather unexpectedly stopped working, and Sareta, just as unexpectedly, was allowed to return to school.

Now there was more friction between grandmother and mother, since Sareta felt that her parents were taking over the baby altogether and closing her out. The grandfather continued to be punitive and unusually strict and once requested that Sareta be removed from his house and placed in foster care before he hurt her. Sareta herself often expressed a wish that this could be done. Twice, a foster home was found for Sareta and Tony, but in the face of this wish becoming a reality, Sareta found reasons both times for not being able to leave her family.

In conferences with her worker, Sareta expressed great ambivalence and confusion about what to do and how she felt. On the one hand, she wanted very much to get out of the house. She was often angry and bitter toward the grandmother for not protecting her against the grandfather's tirades. But she would almost immediately shift to how lonely she would be without the grandmother and her siblings. Prominent among her concerns was how Tony would react to being separated from the grandparents. She realized that he was very attached to them, and she wondered if he would miss them too or be able to tolerate separation from them. She was adamant, however, that she would never "let them have him" if she left home.

Sareta's return to school—her first occasion to be out of the house at all since Tony's birth—occurred at nine months, just at the age when an adverse reaction to separation from his mother might be expected. Although we looked with particular care for some manifestation of such a reaction in this baby, as one possible index of where his primary attachments might lie, we found no change in his behavior, either by family report or our own observation, that could be ascribed to this shift in caretaker arrangements.

The following summer when school was over, Sareta, still not quite 16, was sent out to work from 7:00 AM to 4:00 PM in a cannery. She was still responsible for many household duties, including preparing dinner for the family. Her entire pay was given to her parents. By the end of the summer, Tony's care had been taken over by the grandmother and the rivalry between grandmother and mother increased. However, when school began in the fall, it was Sareta who was reluctant to leave her job to return to school.

But something else was happening during this year and a half. Sareta was no longer a quiet, passive lump of a child, unable to stand up for herself or talk back to her parents. She was becoming more assertive and demanding, especially with the grandmother. At the cannery she had become something of a "pet" of the older women (some as old as 18 or 20) with whom she worked who gave her a great deal of support, education, and attention. Retrospectively, it is clear that this had much to do with her experiments in becoming more independent.

She began to challenge the parental rules: she insisted on having some of her pay for herself, and began to find ways to spend some little time with her former schoolgirl friends. In an act that seemed at once a show of "mothering" her younger sister while opposing her "depriving" mother, she cashed her entire paycheck and bought her sister a much-wished-for coat which the grandmother had refused to buy.

A kind of provocativeness, characteristic of the rebellious adolescent, became more evident. She began to openly use Tony as a threat in her fights with the grandmother, for example, saying she soon would be old enough to leave home and take Tony with her and they would never see him again. Or, conversely, she would say to her, "No, you take care of him. You might as well. He thinks *you* are his mother. Go to 'Mama', Tony." Either gambit was equally effective in raising the red flag.

Now Sareta is 17 and Tony is three. She does not abandon her claim to Tony, nor give up attempts to assert her mothering role. At the same time, she remains very much tied to the grandmother and aware of the grandmother's claim to Tony's affection as well.

At their most recent visit to our unit, Tony performs, as before, slightly above his age level on developmental scales. He has an easy, comfortable relationship with his mother, but there is an odd quality of distance, of self-containment that is unusual in a three year old. He is friendly but low-keyed. He approaches toys with a serious studiousness that is reminiscent of a contractor assessing the work around him that needs to be done. He is the only child we have observed to approach the pounding board with such precision—holding each peg between thumb and finger while pounding it carefully into place.

Tony's grandfather has been seen as the villain throughout this history, and yet we cannot escape the notion that he seems to have given this child the stamp of his identity. It is as if the healthiest and most productive qualities of the grandfather (who is, after all, considered an excellent carpenter) have been integrated by this child into his own more placid and calm personality.

We do not think the problem is over. Sareta, at 17, has become a very pretty girl and for the first time is beginning to date boys. She talks now of her fantasies of setting up her own household, marrying, and having a family of her own. She wants no more babies until she is at least 25 and will never marry anyone who will not take Tony. Whether she lives up to these long-range plans or not, at some point Tony will be split inevitably from one or another of his two "mothers." If he leaves with Sareta when he is six or eight or ten, he will be separated from a large family with many children whom he now regards as siblings in his permanent home. How does he adapt to the separation from them and from the grandparents with whom he has always lived? How will he decide who is his real mother, his real family?

This young mother and this child are fortunate among our sample of very young mothers and their babies in that, however chaotic the family seems to us from the outside, it has provided each of them with stability enough for the development of firm and real object ties. Sareta seems to be well on her way to negotiating her interrupted passage through adolescence, and Tony shows none of the gross defects in ego development that are so evident in Sally or Terry at comparable ages. And yet, no matter what one predicts for the future, it seems unlikely that either will come out unscathed.

DISCUSSION

As we compare our observations and speculations with those of other clinicians, it becomes very clear that some characteristics of our group of young adolescent mothers can be generalized to the characteristics observed by clinicians
working in other inner-city settings. There are, no doubt, other kinds of adolescent mothers, for instance, the suburban population, usually more affluent,
perhaps coming from intact and less chaotic families. We have almost no consistent data nor clinical observations on this group of adolescent mothers other
than isolated individual patients or families seen in clinical psychiatric settings.
Therefore, we must, for the purposes of this chapter, clearly define the population we have studied and indicate that our conclusions regarding the mother-
infant interaction and the shaping of the infants' subsequent object relationships
and ego characteristics derive from our longitudinal clinical observations of this
particular group of adolescent mothers.

In this group of adolescent mothers it is all too plain that socioeconomic
factors weigh heavily upon all aspects of their daily lives, and that frequently the
members of the family are all experiencing deprivation, marginal gratification,
and clear unhappiness in their bonds to one another. Despite the considerable
weight that must be given to the impact of the socioeconomic stress and deprivation, we feel firmly convinced that the more important factors which lead to the
poor adaptation between mother and infant in the early months and to the
infants' later failures of deep-seated capacity for human relationships do not lie
in the socioeconomic stresses, but rather in the intrapsychic forces at work. The
socioeconomic stresses clearly influence and predispose to the heightened impact
of the intrapsychic factors which we speculate are at work in the mother-infant
dyad.

We direct our focus to the specific triad of the infant-mother-grandmother
and feel that, as previously stated, the adolescent mothers we have observed are
not attempting to act out the need for the oedipal child. Rather, the primary
conflict is the struggle for regressive need-fulfillment and the defenses against
such needs. The pregnancy is not so much an expression of oedipal sexual wishes
as it is an expression of the revived preoedipal need to separate and individuate
from the mothering figure.

The overwhelming thrust toward separation and individuation which dominates the earlier phases of any adolescent's life leans on the first experiences of
separation and individuation of toddler life (Mahler et al, 1975; Blos, 1979).

Mahler et al (1975) stated that "phenomenona of normal development can
best be understood when elements of the process are somewhat out of kilter . . .
one is a track of individuation, the evolution of intrapsychic autonomy,
perception, memory, cognition, reality testing; the other is the intrapsychic

developmental track of separation that runs along differentiation, distancing, boundary formation, and disengagement from the mother. . . . The optimal situations seem to be those in which awareness of bodily separation in terms of differentiation from mother goes parallel with (that is to say neither lags far behind nor runs literally far ahead of) the toddler's development of independent autonomous functioning . . . in short, those functions of the ego which serve individuation."

Although in this quotation, the nature of the mother's own separation-individuation attainment is not noted, in the same segment, Mahler commented, "The mother's attitude has to adapt in the entire course of the separation-individuation process—but especially at certain crucial points or crossroads in that process."

It is this necessity which we see compromised in the adolescent mother. Since she has not the internalized experience of her own earliest psychic separation and ego solidarity, she unconsciously fails to resonate with her infant's passage through this phase. Furthermore, she, as an adolescent mother, is now in the throes of her own attempts to recapitulate her earlier individuation struggles. Blos (1979) stated his conviction that "what is in infancy a 'hatching from the symbiotic membrane to become an individuated toddler' (Mahler) becomes in adolescence the shedding of family dependencies, the loosening of infantile object ties in order to become a member of society at large, or simply, of the adult world."

Clearly, the adolescent mother is thrown back into the very dependency which she should and must be trying to relinquish, and, while turning to her own mother for help and support with the baby, unconsciously feels this as an arousal of that earlier dependency which brings with it loss of autonomy and identity.

If there has been incomplete need satisfaction and the internal image of the constant benign love object has been compromised, this second confrontation between opposing internal wishes cannot result in true autonomy and emotional independence. The separation will remain incomplete, intrapsychically represented by longings and defensive patterns of repetition in displacement, or separation by aggressive acts and rejections of the grandmother or her surrogates. This may, indeed, contribute to the extraordinary difficulties in bringing therapeutic interventions to these girl-mothers or in developing a therapeutic alliance with them. The supports and interventions, whether actual or in the form of relationships, may have to be rejected as the disappointing internalized grandmother image is rejected, to substitute for mature separation and attainment of self-esteem. Our clinical observations of abrupt discontinuity in the attention of the girl-mother to her baby, in holding, feeding, soothing—the aggregate of the caregiving behaviors—seem to be indications of the breakthrough of the adolescent's own intense urges for need fulfillment. She wants something for herself at such moments and cannot postpone or delay her clamoring inner demands. The infant's whimpers or screams represent her own inner life too painfully, and she must direct these wishes to the original mothering figure of her own childhood or ward them off with rage and aggression toward the grandmother or displace them to parental substitutes.

In most of the girls we were able to study, the pregnancy itself, that is, the baby as an entity, seemed to be *incidental*, and an attachment to the infant which would lead to the bond between mother and child seemed to be so clouded by the persistent struggle of the girl-mother to separate herself from her own mother that a continuous cathexis of the infant could not be established and maintained. We saw, in a majority of the observations of the mother-infant pairs, that the visual connections between baby and the mother were intermittent and unstable. The babies tended to gaze indiscriminately at other faces or at inanimate objects in the environment.

The adolescent mother was most often in visual contact with the clinical observer or with the grandmother when we observed them in a clinical infant assessment situation or in nondirective interaction. We frequently had the subjective experience that the adolescent mother was attempting to make contact with the clinician or outreach worker, and often simply did not include the infant in her sphere of attention. In one observed period of interaction, the mother did not once take her eyes off the face of the clinician, while all the time holding her baby on her lap with his head dangling over her arm. His frets or whimpers led her to move to jiggle him, but never to look at or soothe him with close, rhythmic cuddling. It was consistently difficult to stimulate the babies to focus and to maintain a fixed gaze. Their visual behavior seemed remarkably similar to the babies who were diagnosed as having failure-to-thrive, even though they were not malnourished or starved-looking. The element of ego and defense formation failure with which we have been most concerned in our later clinical assessments of these babies has been the defective modification of aggressive derivatives. For example, the grandmother who cared for her daughter's 11-month-old baby girl came to us describing Sally as a combination of "hellion and good girl," by which she meant that the alternation between Sally's uncontrollable rage and quiet, receptive, loving periods was unpredictable and unmanageable. This may indicate an identification with the mother's own most prominent conflict during the infant's separation-individuation phase, that is, the mother's docility alternating with rage (however expressed) toward the grandmother.

Most of the adolescent mothers, during the pregnancy and after the birth of the baby, regressed to a more intensely ambivalent tie to the grandmother.

When the adolescent mother and her infant return to the grandparents' home, the baby becomes the center of controversy and the focus of rivalrous confrontation. The mother alternates between her wish to be nurtured as she sees the grandmother nurturing the baby, and her need to possess her infant. It is at this stage we have seen the most regression and revived hostility erupt toward the grandmother from the mother. It is not always in the direct and impulsive form it reached in the Franklin family when Diane draw a knife on her mother, but sometimes in slightly less, but unmistakable, violent manifestations. One mother described actual tugs of war between herself and the grandmother, with the baby between them grabbed and held, or snatched away by the other in these battles. The mother does, in fact, forget about the source of the fight— which has usually been a disagreement over when to feed or where to take the baby—and becomes consciously enraged and filled with longing to have the grandmother cuddle *her*; or she defends against this wish by demanding that the grandmother leave her alone and stop insisting on the rules of the household. Gradually, such primitive ambivalence pushes the grandmother and mother farther apart, and the solution becomes a separation. The baby is likely to be placed in foster care, so that neither triumphs and each member of the triad has lost a crucial love object. But they are then still united in hate toward one another.

We assume that in the early mother-infant dyad the reduction of painful tension and the production of gratification must come from sustained and re-peated interactions between the mother and infant, and that without this gradual cathectic bond the infant will be unable to proceed to actual constancy of object relations and to sustained human intimacy. We also may assume that destructive aggression, while perhaps not adequately understood in its origins, has some deep relationship to the accumulated experiences of frustration and psychic pain within the mother-infant dyad. Some, if not all, of the heightened aggression and hostile destructive impulsivity of the children we have described must then be related to the particular quality of this mother-infant interactional experience.

In two classic papers, Rank (1949) and Rank and MacNaughton (1950), as a part of their description of children with atypical development, delineated a concept of aggressive development that is particularly significant in light of our observations on the children of adolescent mothers. Rank (1949) stated "depri-vation is necessary . . . for the development of the ego, for the differentiation of self and the outside world. However, every transition from indulgence to depri-vation brings tension, which is tolerated only when the child feels secure, confi-dent that indulgence will again follow deprivation. . . . When the mother herself is a poorly organized personality, narcissistic and immature, though not infre-quently extremely conscientious and eager to become a mother, the child's ego has a very precarious existence. It remains largely undifferentiated and hence is not capable of organizing and controlling drives (libidinal and aggressive)." In the later paper, Rank and MacNaughton (1950) enlarged upon this formula-tion, with clinical examples so timely to our own observations that they might have been taken from our own clinical protocols. They speak of the "emotional climate" to denote the subtle and constant aspects of the interaction between mother and child which produce, in large measure, the child's capacity to contain and modulate aggression in response to tension and frustration. The alternation, seen in our sample of adolescent mothers, between excessive fusing behaviors and the abrupt distancing from the babies, lays the internal groundwork for later aggressive attacks against the self or towards others by the child.

The adolescent mother's capacity to feel the infant as the recipient of her giving and soothing care is severely limited by her own sense of wanting to be given to and soothed. Her intermittent and frustration-producing approach sets the stage for both heightened aggression and the lack of a pleasureful bond between the infant and mother. This seems to be responsible for the infant's (and later the toddler's) fixation at a need-fulfillment stage of object relationships, his or her inability to progress to total constancy of human relationships.

The two opposing wishes, dominant in the early adolescent, of a push toward further individuation and a separation from the mother of childhood psychic life, and the breakthrough of regressive longings for fusion and symbiosis with this same pregenital mother, are at their height in the adolescent mother. While we cannot say with certainty, it is compelling to speculate that the pregnancy in the first place neatly represents an attempted solution to both these forces. It is for this reason that most of the adolescent mothers we have seen have not impressed us with the predominance of oedipal structuring, but rather with the continued pressing dyadic nature of their own object ties.

The child does indeed become incidental. Some of the adolescent mothers have been very explicit about this, with comments that they loved the state of pregnancy, feeling full and contented, but began to feel angry and enraged toward the demanding infant once it was not a part of their inner space and needed to be nurtured.

Where there are no modifying forces in the form of supportive maternal figures who can give nurturance to the mother and thereby allow her to cathect the baby with positive and loving feelings, the part-object and aggressive aspects of intrapsychic structure formation seem each to be mutually reinforcing for mothers and babies, producing a developmental trap which is difficult to avoid.

For these children and, often in a mirroring way, for their mothers, the object need is for quick gratification; mother is good only if she instantly relieves tension or pain. The adolescent mother must, because she is caught in a web of her own unmet needs, make a mirror image of her psychic reality in that of her infant. The generational repetition of adolescent motherhood is striking and cannot be simple identification, although we often shorthand the phenomenon descriptively by invoking identification. But the intrapsychic forces are more intricate, and seem to come about as a result of the concatenation of the adolescent struggle to individuate against the wish to regress and fuse, and the infantile need for the totality of maternal preoccupation and need-meeting, which cannot be provided by the adolescent mother. To be the mother of the baby is, then, perhaps an attempt to regain the longed-for mother of the symbiotic phase; but the actuality of attachment and postponement of gratification for the adolescent mother overwhelms her, and the infant cannot become the true object of her nurturance and bonding.

The infant then has a developmental arrest as does her mother. This is found in at least 25 percent of adolescent mothers and in a much higher percentage of the early adolescent mothers (Sugar, 1979).

SUMMARY

We have focused on the problem of the earliest development of object relations experienced by the infants of adolescent mothers and the possible genesis of later failures in the capacity for attainment of constant love objects, with increased aggressive and destructive behaviors which characterize these children. We emphasize that these observations are from our clinical population of inner-city adolescent mothers and suggest that the dynamic triad is one of adolescent mother-grandmother-infant, with   regression in the early adolescent mother to former levels of need wishes directed toward the grandmother. When such earlier stages have been compromised and incomplete, the reemergence of the adolescent mother's prior unfulfilled needs blocks her capacity to constantly cathect and minister to her own infant.

The experiential result for the infant is also a failure to attain sufficient levels of satisfaction and tension reduction over a period of time, thus predisposing to the inconstant nature of later object relationships and the dominance of aggressive and hostile responses to love objects in later developmental phases.

We have noted the circumscribed nature of our clinical population—that is, inner-city adolescent mothers, for whom socioeconomic pressures are constantly a part of life experience. However, we feel that the primary dynamic issues are internal and are located in the early phases of infant-mother interaction, shadowed and mirrored by the mother's own incomplete need satisfaction and revived in her early adolescent yearnings.

REFERENCES

Blos, P. 1979. *The Adolescent Passage: Developmental Issues.* New York: International Universities Press, pp. 141-170.
Edgecumbe, R. and Bergner, M. 1972. Some problems in the conceptualization of early object relationships. I: The concepts of need satisfaction and need satisfying relationships. II: The concept of object constancy. *Psychoanal. Study Child* 27:283-314, 315-333.

Lichtenberg, J. D. 1975. The development of the sense of self. *J. Am. Psycho-anal. Assoc.* 23:453–484.

Mahler, M., Pine, F. and Bergman, A. 1975. *The Psychological Birth of the Human Infant: Symbiosis and Individuation.* New York: Basic Books, pp. 55–64.

Rank, B. 1949. Aggression. *Psychoanal. Study Child* 3/4:43–48.

Rank, B. and MacNaughton, D. 1950. A clinical contribution to early ego development. *Psychoanal. Study Child* 5:53–65.

Sugar, M. 1979. Developmental aspects of adolescent motherhood. In M. Sugar (Ed.): *Female Adolescent Development.* New York: Brunner/Mazel.

Weil, A. 1972. The basic core. *Psychoanal. Study Child* 25:442–460.

Some Current Programs
for Adolescent Parenthood

9

Preparing Adolescents in Child Bearing: Before and After Pregnancy

NICHOLAS ANASTASIOW

INTRODUCTION

The art of successful parenting has been well established by millions of individuals across the world. It appears that facilitating parenting skills are practiced by a variety of racial and ethnic groups and are not the exclusive province of the white middle class (Schachter, 1979; Werner et al, 1971; Werner, 1980). Parents are able to facilitate their children's development so that as infants, they achieve their developmental milestones; as children they manage the social and academic demands of school; and as adults they are able to fulfill Freud's dictum of maturity—the ability to work and love. These parents have come to learn that infants do not develop solely on their own due to the process of genetically determined maturation. These parents seem to know that infants require an environment which is responsive to their needs and a caregiver who encourages them to make developmental advances (Kearsley, 1979; Zelazo, 1979).

Many parents in the United States are knowledgeable about and practice what we refer to as facilitating parenting techniques. These techniques include the caregiver's responding to the child's attempt to understand and cope with the world, providing verbal stimulation to and vocal games for the child's own attempts at verbalization, establishing an atmosphere of warmth and acceptance, stimulating the child's cognitive development, and pressing the child to make developmental advances (Hunt, 1979). In Wertheim's (1975) sense, the successful caregiver assists the child in the development of both autonomy and competence. Furthermore, these facilitating parenting skills have been shown to advance children's language development, verbal and nonverbal IQ scores, and general social adjustment in schools, and are related to the child's school completion and employability (Werner et al, 1971; Werner and Smith, 1977; Bradley and Caldwell, 1978; Bradley et al, 1979).

In fact, these parenting skills are so instrumental in aiding development that infants who suffer trauma at birth, such as anoxia or breech birth, have a better chance of overcoming the trauma if the primary caregivers utilize these facilitating techniques (Werner et al, 1971; Sameroff, 1979). The effects of the nature of the caregiver's childrearing practices are so powerful that Broman and associates (1975) of the National Collaborative Longitudinal Study have concluded that anoxia and breech birth are trivial in comparison to what it is a caregiver does in the home with an infant and child.

Unfortunately, for a large segment of the world's population (many of whom reside in unfavorable economic conditions), facilitating parenting techniques are not performed routinely. Devitalizing attitudes toward children still persist. These include the high use of physical punishment, low verbalization, a laissez-faire attitude toward achievement of developmental milestones, and low expression of affection. This set of attitudes has been shown to have a debilitating effect on verbal and cognitive development (Werner and Smith, 1977; Bradley and Caldwell, 1978).

In the Werner and colleagues (1971) study, perinatal stress factors were magnified by the unaffectionate, low stimulating homes to such a degree that each child in the low socioeconomic status (SES), low stimulation group was seen as having a school problem at age ten; many had below normal IQs. Perinatal stress seems to be related to a variety of handicapping conditions at school age when accompanied by low facilitating parenting practices (Werner and Smith, 1977; Sameroff, 1979). These negative effects are further confounded when the parent who administers them also resides in poverty (Werner, 1980).

Given the results of these studies, it would appear that the effect of parenting techniques should be widely disseminated along with details of the facilitating practices so as to enhance the quality of life for yet unborn infants.

It is the basic premise of this chapter that efforts to equip future parents with these facilitating techniques should be a basic part of each young person's education. Educational programs that focus on normal child growth and development and the caregiver techniques that facilitate development are needed to insure that each normal infant reaches his genetic potential and that each infant born at risk may overcome it. Such programs are critically needed today due to the fact that the segment of the world's young people are not trained in or aware of child development needs are bearing children at alarming rates (Bogue, 1977). Thousands of young people ten to 16 years of age who have not learned the facilitative strategies of child rearing are becoming parents each year. The infants of these adolescent parents are at greater physiological risk, tend to make slower developmental gains, suffer a greater amount of psychological and physiological abuse, and are at greater sociological risk (see Chapters 7 and 8, this volume).

The variety of educational programs described in this chapter have been established to train these young parents to effectively raise their children, and to assist the mother in assuming the social-psychological responsibility of parenthood. As we shall see below, programs vary in their basic goals and the settings in which the intervention is carried out. Some programs attempt to treat the mother while she is pregnant or just after the birth of her child. Other programs concentrate on family planning, which encourages birth control procedures and discourages early childbearing. A growing number of programs focus on teaching child development and child rearing techniques in junior, middle, and senior high schools. Each type of program will be examined in turn. First we will examine the standard view maintained by schools toward teenage pregnancies.

EARLY PROGRAMS FOR PREGNANT TEENAGERS

Before the national increase in births to teenagers, it was a common custom to ask a girl to leave regular school if she became pregnant. In some cases, the girl was provided with a home teacher and was able to continue the academic work of the school. In many communities, the girl was not encouraged to return to regular school after the birth of her child and was frequently perceived as immoral and a bad influence on the other students. The exclusions were supported by the communities' values and standards (Washington, 1975).

As the teenage birth rate accelerated in the 1950s and 1960s, a rash of programs for pregnant teenagers was established in the larger urban centers. The urban areas with dense population felt the impact of the large numbers of pregnancies early while rural areas experienced the same percent increase but had a smaller total number of pregnant girls. Some of these early programs still exist but many disappeared as government funds became unavailable.

During the 1960s, alliances such as the National Alliance Concerned with School-Age Parents (Eddinger, 1977) and their state alliances, such as California and Oregon, encouraged the establishment of alternative classes and schools for the pregnant girl. In many communities, such as Gary, Indiana, the young girl could attend an alternative class with other pregnant girls and maintain her academic program. In some cases, additional information on child care was added to the course of study. In a limited number of cities, such as New York, alternative classes were made available, but pregnant girls were also allowed to remain in their regular classes, a practice which continues today. The majority of most recently established programs allow the girl to remain with her peers (Bolton, 1980).

The major focus of these classes was on maintaining the regular school program and introducing some notions of child care and home management. In essence, the classes were unsuccessful and most pregnant girls dropped out of school after delivery of their infant. Further, many of these girls had a repeat pregnancy within a year and a third child before the age of 20. In a few cities, alternative programs out of the school were designed "to treat" the girl. In one type, attempts were made to deal with the psychodynamically perceived dilemmas of the young adolescent and their perceived "problem" in desiring to have an infant during the teenage period.

In virtually all of these early writings, the girl is seen to be "sick" and in need of treatment. Almost all of these efforts focused on "the problem" of the pregnancy and dealt exclusively with the girl and not the (father) boy. Rarely was the girl's pregnancy seen as a product of a cultural epoch in which she might have been the victim.

Documentation of the results of these early programs is almost nonexistent. Schools responded to the growing number of pregnancies and in almost all cases did not evaluate program effectiveness on the girl, on high school completion, on future pregnancies, or on any other dimension. As harsh as it may sound, the schools can be perceived as wishing the problem would go away. In the main, the girls who became pregnant were dealt with as immoral outcasts. It was not the schools alone who viewed the girls as guilty. A similar position by health care professionals has been described by Abbott (1977). Abbott's work involved the training of health care professionals in breaking down the negative reactions they had toward the sexually active teenagers. It has been difficult for professionals and lay personnel alike to conceptualize that children from the ages of ten to 15 were sexually active. As the number of pregnancies increased, attitudes began to change and new efforts were initiated.

COMPREHENSIVE SCHOOL PROGRAMS

The combined results of earlier sexual maturation by both males and females and the increasing number of sexually active teenagers led to the commonly referred to one million pregnancies and 600,000 live births to teenagers (Anastasiow et al, 1978). It should be noted that the most common location for conception is in the girl's home after school (Whitelaw, Personal Communication, 1980). Also of importance is the fact that teenagers of the same age are engaging in sexual intercourse, which is contrary to the myth of an older boy engaging in sexual intercourse with a much younger girl. Evidence from several countries indicates that adolescents are in general not promiscuous (Engstrom, 1978). The relationship established among the couples appears to be a lasting one in which sex partners are maintained over a period of time. Kinch and Kruger (1970) suggested that less than 22 percent of sexually active teen-agers change partners over a one-year period of time. The lower age of sexual maturation has affected both sexes. Both sexes mature and are sexually active at a younger age (Anastasiow et al, 1974). These factors place unique demands on those family planners who may be faced with young parents who might both be 14 years of age or younger. Many agencies became involved in the issue and pressed schools "to do something." Many communities and states resisted teaching about contraception but others began to modify their school organization and programs to respond to adolescent pregnancy; still others added family planning information into the curriculum, as was the case in New York City.

In the late 1960s, a few communities established comprehensive school programs that attempted to provide a broad range of health and academic services. Of special note are the McCabe Center in New Haven (Holmes et al, 1970; Foltz et al, 1972), and the Educational Services for School Age Parents in New Brunswick, New Jersey (Bennett and Bardon, 1977), Maryland (Dohrmann, 1979), and California (Stine and Kelley, 1970). Some of these programs were located in facilities that were separate from the normal school (See a description of the Hill Health Center, Chapter 11, this volume).

A strong educational program by Planned Parenthood was launched to make contraceptive information available to teenagers. The dispensation of contraceptives existed mostly outside of the school. At least two programs were established in a regular school which dispensed contraceptives, one in Washington, DC and the other in St. Paul, Minnesota (Marmet, 1977; Alton, 1979). These programs offered a wide range of services, including response to the adolescent's emotional as well as medical concerns. A recent report suggests that there was a major reduction in pregnancies when these programs were placed into a comprehensive framework such as the St. Paul program, which is discussed in more detail later (Alton, 1979; Edwards et al, 1980). However, many writers noted that teenagers' sense of cause-effect and probability is poorly developed and before the first pregnancy they are unresponsive to contraceptive use (Bogue, 1977; Zabin et al, 1979; Chapter 7, this volume).

These comprehensive programs generally attempted to maintain the regular academic program or provide alternate vocational training. Health counseling and medical and social services were available, usually with the cooperation of a local clinic or hospital. These schools reported success in maintaining the girl in school during pregnancy, returning to graduate after delivery, and in improving a number of infant and maternal health factors (Holmes et al, 1970; Foltz et al 1972; Bennett and Bardon, 1977; Osofsky and Osofsky, 1970; Dohrmann, 1979; Stine and Kelley, 1970). In some cases, the high schools established preschool centers to which the mother brought her infant while she continued high school (Stine and Kelley, 1970).

Let us examine the St. Paul program (Alton, 1979) more closely as an example of what a comprehensive program could be.

The St. Paul program operated in two schools which were junior-senior high schools. The groundwork for establishing the program was arduous, with many parents objecting to the dispensing of contraceptives in the school. However, the school board approved it unanimously, provided the program did not interfere with the regular academic program. To begin with, the first dispensing of contraceptives took place in an evening adolescent clinic in a neighboring hospital. The second dispensing center was an abandoned school closet, and eventually a fully equipped center was established within the school.

In full operation it included pre- and postnatal care, veneral disease testing and treatment, pregnancy testing, Pap smears, and information and counseling on contraceptive use (Edwards et al, 1980).

The personnel in the clinic who provided the pregnancy tests also initiated the family planning needs with the young girl and boy. The boy was included if he was identified as the father after the pregnancy of the girl was determined. As the clinic expanded, the services were enlarged to include physicals for athletic, occupational, and college needs as well as immunizations. Edwards and associates (1980) believed the expansion of the clinic to include more than pregnancy and contraceptive information made the clinic more desirable to a wider range of students and provided some anonymity for the sexually active teenager.

Family planning courses contained information on prenatal care, human sexuality, parenting, and the roles and responsibility of family members. (One topic was the "First Years of a Baby's Life.")

The authors reported that the emotional concerns of the adolescent were attended to by social workers and/or other relevant professionals. The St. Paul program also provided obstetric and nutritional counseling, a dental hygienist, and a day care center. The day care center provided child care while the adolescent parents completed high school. The infants received cognitive and emotional stimulation in the day care center while their parents, both fathers and mothers, received training in the center.

We can find little in the literature that directly addresses the problem of how to assist very young parents assume the responsibility of parenthood. The author is aware of a case in Ohio in which two 12 year olds were married to legitimize an impending birth. Marriage was the only solution acceptable to the religious parents of both of the youngsters.

In most program descriptions, the case studies concern older adolescents, 16 or 17, who are potentially able to assume the roles of marriage, family, and parenthood. Yet to be discovered is how programs can address the needs of a modern-day Romeo and Juliet. The poignant description of a 14-year-old Puerto Rican mother of a newborn in New York City whose 13-year-old lover leaves her for another 14 year old is to many a horror story, with abortion thought to be the only sane solution (Clinef, 1979).

Although many comprehensive programs are designed for both sexes, most exist in high school and deal with older adolescents.

The success of programs, such as that in St. Paul, in reducing pregnancy and obstetric complications and in establishing a vocational orientation among students, has encouraged the establishment of other comprehensive centers; however, these programs focus on a small bit of the complex issue of adolescent pregnancy. The data suggest that there are 6.9 million sexually active male teenagers in the United States, with many of the males having first intercourse at age 12. The number of sexually active females may be as high as 40 percent of the 15 to 19-year-old group, with an estimated 375,000 sexually active females of 13 to 14 years of age (Bolton, 1980).

In addition, a growing number of young girls are electing to keep their babies and not to give the child up for adoption. In the large urban areas, many of these young girls leave their families and set up separate residences of their own. Thus, the burden of adequately raising the infant falls to the young mother, who is often alone and does not have her own emotional needs being met by a parent or husband. While the total proportion of teenage births in proportion to the teenage population is decreasing, illegitimacy has increased (Dryfoos, 1978). Thus, the problem is double-edged. Programs must be designed to care for the emotional needs of the young mother as well as the needs of her infant.

PROGRAMS IN HOSPITALS AND CLINICS

In the absence of concentrated efforts by schools and communities, hospital personnel were faced with a large number of children bearing children. As has been stated, medical personnel did not always know how to respond to the sexually active teenager and usually did so in a "good-bad" continuum (Abbott, 1977). Thus hospitals were faced with responding to, or ignoring, the problem of the increased number of teenage births. Hospital and clinic personnel rarely had an opportunity to reach young people before they became pregnant (Graham, 1977).

The author is personally familiar with a city hospital that was overwhelmed with a large number of teenage births and closed the obstetric service of the hospital. This placed enormous demands on the remaining hospital in the community. The two educational nurses of the hospital found their services directed away from the training of heart and stroke patients in an attempt to prevent teenage pregnancies. The hospital readily cooperated with a parenting program for junior high school youngsters when approached.

Although very few of the hospitals attempted to assist the adolescent parent in coping with the responsibilities of parenthood, one outstanding example of a hospital that desired to assist the young parent on a broad set of dimensions can be seen in the program designed by Badger (1979) in Cincinnati. This program was developed at the request of the hospital staff in response to the large number of children born to teenage parents in the hospital. Badger and her coworkers contact the young mother in the hospital soon after the birth of her child. They believe that the young girl is susceptible to respond positively to learning how to care for her infant during this period. They wish to teach the mother techniques that will intensify the mother's competence and satisfaction in rearing her child. The mother is taught how to interact with her baby, respond to the infant's verbal behavior, encourage play, and teach developmental skills.

The results are very encouraging for the more than 800 mothers who have been trained. Their babies' IQ scores are normal compared with the offspring of untrained teenage mothers whose mean IQ score is 79. In contrast to the bleak national picture of the untreated adolescent mother being on welfare and having another child within a year, Badger's group tends to have fewer second children; two thirds are employed and some have returned to school. The Cincinnati program appears to do what it aims to do, that is, to mobilize the mother's resources at a critical time, enabling her to effectively deal with herself and her infant.

Similar results have been achieved by other hospital- or clinic-based interventions on San Francisco by Goldstein et al (1973) and in Texas by Smith and associates (1978) (see Chapter 10, this volume). Abbott (1977) and Graham (1977) noted the positive impact of their training procedures at Columbia-Presbyterian Hospital in New York. Grady (1975) described a comprehensive medical center-maternity home program which focused on the wide range of health and academic needs. This program attempts to include fathers as well. In addition, many of the hospital programs provide follow-up counseling and assistance (Smith et al 1978). Some attempts to contact adolescents before pregnancy through a "hotline" for adolescents providing information on birth control have been established in the United States and in other countries (Smith et al 1975; Sanchez, 1977).

A variation of the hospital-based program is the one of Field and associates (1979) in Florida, which is a home-based program for the new mother on a biweekly basis. They reported positive effects of the program on infant and mother. Of interest is the higher blood pressure reading of the trained mothers; these investigators conjectured that training may result in increasing the mother's anxiety about her infant's progress.

There are innumerable efforts at training parents how to raise their children (Gordon et al, 1975; Hanes et al, 1976). Many of these efforts grew out of the poverty programs such as Head Start, which mandated parent involvement (Zigler and Valentine, 1979). The variety of programs training parents increased with the spread of preschool programs for handicapped youngsters developed under the Early Childhood Handicapped Program Assistance Act (DeWeerd, 1974). These programs are not exclusively designed for adolescent parents but do contain many young parents in their population.

The popularity of training parents to effectively raise or remediate their child's deficit in case of impairment has grown (Wiegerink and Parrish, 1975). One recent development is the establishment of the Betty Phillip's Center for Parenthood Education at Peabody College, Vanderbilt University, in Nashville, Tennessee. One of the major goals of the center is to train teachers who would instruct in the parenthood courses in secondary schools.

An interesting variation is the "Parent-Infant Support Through Lay Health Visitors" program operating in Denver. This program provides trained lay personnel to mothers 16 years and over, in midpregnancy through the baby's first year of life. The lay personnel are experienced mothers who have been trained and are under the supervision of a public health nurse. The home visitors attempt to enhance family stability and parenting skills. A strong emphasis was made on the needs of the infant and ways to facilitate the infant's social adjustment and cognitive growth (van Doorninck et al, 1980).

In essence, the comprehensive school and hospital programs "treat" the mother and infant. They appear to be able to improve the life chances and environments of both. The services are multidisciplinary, include health, academic, occupational, and child care training and counseling, and are aimed at adolescents who reside in low socioeconomic conditions. The intervention is as much social as it is medical, aiming to improve the mother's life and thereby her child's. In some cases, it reduces the number of repeat pregnancies. However, in spite of all of these efforts, teenage pregnancies are still occurring. In our opinion, these programs are highly desirable and should be continued, but many are still medical-model oriented. That is, they, "treat problems" rather than educate for primary prevention.

CHILD DEVELOPMENT PROGRAMS

The next group of programs discussed is primary prevention—these seek to expose young people to the full array of children's developmental needs and to the responsibility of parenthood *before* they become parents.

Child development has been taught traditionally by the home economics department of the junior and senior high schools. However, many of these programs reach only a small proportion of the students in junior or senior high school. A rare exception is the program in Texas which is broad-based, and includes family living, child development, and work study and laboratory

training in child development. In addition, a large number of boys are attracted
to the Texas program, whereas most home economic courses include only girls
(Education Commission of the States, 1975).

Probably the most widely adopted program is Education for Parenthood
(Morris, 1977) which was developed as a cooperative effort of Administration
for Children, Youth and Families, the US Office of Education, and the National
Institute of Mental Health. The program is designed to provide classroom instruction in child development and practicum experience with young children.
The curriculum was designed to present a course in child development that
would include the social, medical, and emotional needs of children, the family's
role in socialization, the important factors in prenatal care and early infancy,
and child care career possibilities (Morris, 1977). The program is being used in
over 5,000 schools and several hundred colleges and universities, community
agencies, and foreign sites.

This program is designed for senior high school as a one-year elective
course. The curriculum combines classroom study with field-site experience
in early child care settings such as Head Start, day care centers, and parent
cooperatives. In some cases, the early childhood class is located in the high
school and contains children of high school students.

In an expansion of the program, seven national voluntary youth organ-
izations were involved in developing parenthood education in nonschool settings.
These voluntary organizations included the Boy Scouts of America, the Boy's
Club of America, National 4-H Club, Foundation of America, Girl Scouts of
the USA, National Federation of Settlements and Neighborhood Centers, the
Salvation Army, and Save the Children Federation.

One of the major strengths of the program is the well designed curriculum
called "Exploring Childhood." The material was extensively tested in the field
and is cf high quality design and content. The curriculum contains films, film-
strips, books, pamphlets, and an excellent teacher guide, teacher training
materials, and a guide for the school administrator. Development of materials
was supported by federal and private (March of Dimes) funds. The Education
Development Center of Massachusetts distributes the materials. Little data
are available to evaluate the impact of the course of study on adolescent pregnancy or childrearing. The available data suggest small but positive gains in
knowledge, attitudes, and skills among the participants of the regular high
school program (Cobb and Peters, 1975; von Hippel and Cohen, 1976) and
similar small but positive gains in the outreach programs (Morris, 1977).

Montgomery County (Maryland) schools offer a year-long course in the
senior high that involves students in laboratory as well as in class activities.
The "labs" are located in the high school and are attended by preschoolers
from the community. The high school student observes, plans lessons, and
interacts with young children. Several thousand students have participated
in this experience (Education Commission of the States, 1975).

Both the Montgomery County and Exploring Childhood courses are perceived as offering valuable experience with young children as well as providing the adolescent with the opportunity to gain insight into his/her own feelings and desires.

As desirable as the Exploring Childhood and Montgomery County courses are, considering the drop-out rate of the pregnant teenager during junior high school, the developers of FEED (Facilitating Environments Encouraging Development) argued that programs are offered too late for many adolescents (Anastasiow and associates, 1978). FEED was designed for junior and middle high school female and male students. The program utilizes curriculum developed by others, such as Exploring Childhood. The developers extensively reviewed multimedia materials in the area of child development and determined the suitability of the materials for the 11 to 14 year old. A set of comprehensive objectives for a child development course was developed to key multimedia teaching material to each objective. A coordinator's guide has been developed for school and/or community leaders for guidance in developing a local FEED program.

The basic intent of FEED is to prepare young people, *before* they become parents, in principles of child growth and development, particularly parenting skills that facilitate development. FEED's educational philosophy assumes that the student is the active learner and that activities should be designed to involve the student in an active interchange. Thus, classroom experiences alone were perceived as being an inadequate vehicle for delivering curriculum, which includes not only knowledge and skills but attitudes toward infants and young children and attitudes toward the responsibility of parenting. FEED provides three practicum sites: a health care facility, an early childhood center for normal children, and a child care center for handicapped children. It attempts to have the students (boys and girls) serve as teachers and aides to children in these centers so that they can confront their own attitudes toward infants and young children, discover the source of some handicapping conditions related to early childbearing, and discover the services offered by all three centers.

The data to date suggest that the FEED program has a pronounced impact on the students' attitudes and knowledge concerning normal and handicapped children. Follow-up study of the long-term effects of FEED is underway. Based on the FEED experience and the reviews of the literature, the following suggestions are offered on program effectiveness.

DESIRABLE CHARACTERISTICS OF EDUCATIONAL PROGRAMS

This chapter is based on the assumption that adolescents will continue to bear and parent a substantial number of infants each year. In order to prepare these young people for this; a child development course at the junior and intermediate level is but one attempt to introduce the students to the responsibilities of parenthood. However, programs should operate at several levels and focus on child growth and development.

Many communities are resistent to the teaching of contraceptive use (the state of Oklahoma for example), but this need not stop the teaching of child development and parenting skills. It is our opinion that the seventh grade is an excellent place to begin for several reasons. First of all most of the students have undergone or are undergoing earlier sexual maturation (Anastasiow et al, 1974). Most adolescent sexual experimentation has the potential consequence of pregnancy due to the early physiologic maturation of boys and girls. Whereas in prior generations, if early sexual play involved two young people, one of them was probably physiologically immature. Even though a young girl in the 1930 generation had menarche at 14 she would not have ovulated until she was 16. For the boy, the age in drop in voice has been documented since the time of Johann Sebastian Bach (Roche, 1979). Today's boys experience a voice drop four years earlier than Bach's choir boys, but little or no data are available in the relationship of sperm count and voice drop. Possibly, boys' fertility has a parallel in girls', that is, a one- or two-year lag between voice drop and sperm virility. Some authors have speculated that the "real" sexual revolution in the United States occurred during the 1919--1929 period (Bolton, 1980). The increase in numbers of sexually active teenagers was steady, with a growing acceptance of intercourse as a personal choice by high school students in the 1960s and 1970s. The lower age of maturation and the increased acceptance of premarital intercourse has created a situation that society has not yet fully faced.

As Smith (Chapter 10, this volume) indicates, the majority of sexually active adolescents are normal and do not wish to delay their sexual life. The societies in the world that wish to control for adolescent sexuality outside of marriage, provide for and encourage early marriage (Deschamps and Valantin, 1978).

Secondly, 12 to 14 year olds are open to experience and are in the main cut out of the main work force of the community. Most states have work laws prohibiting these young people's inclusion in community agencies. Lipsitz (1977) described this period of life as "Growing Up Forgotten." Junior and senior high schools are bleak institutions to many adolescents. In the opinion of many, there are few meaningful things for these students to do and the young adolescent responds gratefully to being needed. Kubie (1959) noted from his long-term observations that those persons who had developed a sense of compassion had an opportunity as adolescents to experience suffering *and* had an opportunity to minister to it. Further, adolescence is a period of rapid change of physical, cognitive, and social values (Conger, 1977). As Conger noted, the complexity of the adolescent period has attracted the attention of our major developmental theorists including Freud, Erikson, Piaget, and Bandura. It's a period of isolation in which the adolescent turns to peers for advice, comfort, and satisfaction of needs. The pregnancy issue is embedded in a web of developmental issues in which each strand of the web stands out in the morning dew and has been dealt with separately by society.

In our opinion, it is critical that young teenagers have such an out-of-school opportunity; the practicum experience in working with handicapped children in FEED is one such experience. Other meaningful experiences need to be invented to engage the adolescent in a full use of his capacities.

The practicum site allows adolescents to confront their own feelings regarding childbearing, child rearing, and handicapped children. In one FEED site the FEED students, saddened, and grieving over the death of a three year old in the hospital, were able to work out these emotions with the adults in that setting. They became very angry and judgmental about the child's mother, who at age 13 had given birth to the child and abandoned the child. The FEED students were able to express these emotions and receive help in developing their own attitudes toward early pregnancy. Other FEED students have discovered their dislike for infants and have been helped by the adult in the setting to accept these feelings as "normal" for that person.

Third, the 10 to 14 year old child's attitudes are undergoing examination and are susceptible to change. The teenage period has been recognized as major for the questioning of attitudes and values. As Piaget has noted, it is a period when all values are subject to question and any possibility is seen as probable no matter how unique (Elkind, 1978).

Fourth, some of these 12 and 13 year olds may become parents before the year is out. We believe programs begun in the seventh grade should continue in some form throughout the junior and senior high school years, perhaps at seventh, ninth, and 11th grades. The program should be a community effort and include many disciplines. Child care centers can serve as practicum or work study sites. Health care facilities can serve as models of desirable health care. In the health care facility, the junior or senior high student is a valuable resource in reading stories or interacting with long-term patients who are children. Such facilities expose the junior or senior high students to the range of health services provided but also to a range of occupational and professional models. FEED personnel found that this exposure tended to break down fears of health care workers held by junior high students and improved the students' overall attitude towards adults.

The child development course should be oriented toward what can be accomplished by a facilitating child care technique. Too frequently, the courses for pregnant teenagers have perceived the pregnant girl as a problem rather than as a girl with a new set of responsibilities and needs. Viewing the issue from a psychopathologic basis appears to have little utility (Bolton, 1980).

The program must be multidisciplinary and include teachers, psychologists, social workers, psychiatrists, and other health care professionals. However, the programs cannot be effective unless community values and attitudes towards the sexually active adolescent remain positive (Chapter 10, this volume). A child development course is but one element in the need of the young. There is a wide range of human needs that are not being provided for in the adolescent in today's society, a subject far too lengthy to be dealt with here, and far too little understood from lack of substantive research (Chapter 7, this volume).

Adolescents in turn need to see the role that they can play as responsible citizens in a society. One of these roles is parenthood. These future parents need a broad exposure to the demands, responsibilities, and, hopefully, the joys of parenthood.

SUMMARY

Early childbearing is the result of a complex set of genetic and social issues. Human sexuality is a strong force traditionally controlled by family members in most countries of the world through the enforcement of abstinence (Deschamps and Valantin, 1978). With the breakdown of the family, throughout the world from urbanization, the sexual activity of the young members of the society has less societal control, and given its genetic force tends to express itself at younger ages. Only a few countries, such as China, are still successful in enforcing sexual abstinence among its members before marriage. Given the younger physiologic maturation of both sexes, these expressions of sexuality are resulting in large numbers of teenage pregnancies.

This chapter has discussed examples of programs designed to respond to teenage sexuality. As we have seen, some programs attempt to prevent pregnancy by dispensing contraceptive devices and encouraging their use. Other programs attempt to train the young mother, and father if available, in how to raise their infant. Exploring Childhood and FEED are two examples of programs designed for students that focus on both sex and the students' mastery of knowledge of child development and parenting skills. Both programs assume that all students can benefit from a course in child development.

No one program is viewed as more desirable than another, although the comprehensive programs described tend to provide for a set of adolescent needs. Much more needs to be done. Too many communities appear to believe that sexuality is encouraged if it is discussed. Rather, in those communities in which human sexuality is discussed, a number of benefits accrue to the community and to the young people for whom the programs are designed, such as reduction of teenage pregnancies, the reduction of low birth weight and premature babies, and the acquisition of healthy attitudes toward the responsibility of child-bearing and child rearing by the population of future parents.

REFERENCES

Abbott, M.I. 1977. *The Teen is Pregnant: What Happens Now?* Presented at The Public Health Association, 108th Annual Convention, Los Angeles, California.

Alton, I.R. 1979. Nutrition services for pregnant adolescents within a public high school. *J. Am. Diet. Assoc.* 74:667–669.

Anastasiow, N.J., Everett, M., O'Shaughnessy, T.E., Eggleston, P.J., and Eklund, S.J. 1978. Using a child development curriculum to change young teen-agers' attitudes toward children, handicapping conditions and hospital settings. *Am. J. Orthopsychiatry* 48(4):663–672.

Anastasiow, N.J., Grimmett, S.A., Eggleston, P.J., and O'Shaughnessy, T.E. 1974. Educational implications of earlier sexual maturation. *Phi Delta Kappan* 26(3):198–200.

Badger, E. 1979. *Effects of Parent Education Program on Teenage Mothers and Their Offspring.* Presented at the International Workshop on the "At-Risk" Infant, Tel Aviv, Israel, July 1979.

Bennett, V.C., and Bardon, J.I. 1977. The effects of a school program on teen-age mothers and their children. *Am. J. Orthopsychiatry* 47:671–678.

Bogue, D.J. (Ed.). 1977. *Adolescent Fertility: The Proceedings of an International Conference.* Chicago, Illinois: Community and Family Study Center, University of Chicago.

Bolton, F.G. Jr. 1980. *The Pregnant Adolescent: Problems of Premature Parenthood.* Beverly Hills, California: Sage Publications.

Bradley, R.H., Caldwell, B.M., and Elardo, R. 1979. Home environment and cognitive development in the first 2 years: a cross-lagged panel analysis. *Dev. Psych.* 15(3):246–250.

Bradley,R.H., and Caldwell, B.M. 1978. Screening the environment. *Am. J. Orthopsychiatry* 48(1):114–130.

Broman, S.H., Nichols, P.L., and Kennedy, W.A. 1975. *Preschool IQ.* Hillsdale, New Jersey: Lawrence Erlbaum Associates.

Clinef, F.X. 1979. The children of desire. *New York Times,* September 30, pp. 14–18.

Cobb, C.M. and Peters, E. 1975. *Summary of Evaluation Findings, Year One.* Cambridge, Massachusetts: Education Development Center.

Conger, J.J. 1977. *Adolescence and Youth: Psychological Development in a Changing World.* New York: Harper & Row.

DeWeerd, J. 1974. Federal programs for the handicapped. *Except. Child.* 40(6):441.

Deschamps, J.P. and Valantin, A. 1978. Pregnancy in adolescence: incidence and outcome in European countries. In A.S. Parker, R.V. Short, M. Potts and M.A. Herbertson (Eds.): *Fertility in Adolescence.* Cambridge, England: Galton Foundation, pp. 101–116.

Dohrmann, H. 1979. Nutrition education in the Santa Ana teen mother program. *J. Am. Diet. Assoc.* 74:665–667.

Dryfoos, G. 1978. The incidence and outcome of adolescent pregnancy in the United States. In A.S. Parker, R.V. Short, M. Potts and M.A. Herbertson (Eds.): *Fertility in Adolescence.* Cambridge, England: Galton Foundation, pp. 85–100.

Eddinger, L. 1977. Helping school-age parents in rural communities. Washington, DC: National Alliance Concerned with School-Age Parents. Pamphlet #301-654-2335.

Education Commission of the States. 1975. *The Role of the Family in Child Development: Implications for State Policies and Programs.* The 15th report of the Education of the States, Early Childhood Project. Denver, Colorado: Education Commission of the States.

Edwards, L.E., Steinman, M.E., Arnold, K.A. and Hakanson, E.Y. 1980. Adolescent pregnancy prevention services in high school clinics. *Fam. Plann. Perspect.* 12(1):6–14.

Elkind, D. 1978. *The Child's Realith: Three Developmental Themes.* Hillsdale, New Jersey: LEA Publishers.

Engstrom, L. 1978. Teenage pregnancy in developing countries. In A.S. Parker, R.V. Short, M. Potts and M.A. Herbertson (Eds.): *Fertility in Adolescence.* Cambridge, England: Galton Foundation, pp. 117–128.

Field, T., Widmayer, S., Stringer, S. and Ignatoff, E. 1979. *An Intervention and Developmental Follow-Up of Preterm Infants Born to Teenage, Lower Class Mothers.* Presented at the International Workshop on the "At Risk" Infant, Tel Aviv, Israel, July 1979.

Foltz, A.M., Klerman, L.V. and Jekel, J.F. 1972. Pregnancy and special education: who stays in school? *Am. J. Publ. Health* 62:1612–1619.

Goldstein, P.J., Zalar, M.K., Grady, E.W. and Smith, R.W. 1973. Vocational education: an unusual approach to adolescent pregnancy. *J. Reprod. Med.* 10:77–79.

Gordon, I.J., Hanes, M., Lamme, L. and Schlenker, P., with the assistance of Barnett, H. 1975. *Parent Oriented Home-Based Early Childhood Education Programs: A Decision Oriented Review.* Gainesville, Florida: Institute for Development of Human Resources, College of Education, University of Florida, May 30, 1975.

Grady, E.W. 1975. Models of comprehensive service-hospital based. *J. School Health* 45:268.

Graham, E. 1977. Medical responsibilities. In D.J. Bogue (Ed.): *Adolescent Fertility: The Proceedings of an International Conference.* Chicago, Illinois: Community and Family Study Center, University of Chicago.

Hanes, M., Gordon, I. and Breivogel, W. (Eds.). 1976. *Update: The First Ten Years of Life.* Proceedings from the Conference Celebrating the Tenth Anniversary of the Institute for Development of Human Resources. Gainesville, Florida: College of Education, University of Florida, March 1976.

Holmes, M.E., Klerman, L.V. and Gabrielson, I.W. 1970. A new approach to educational services for the pregnant student. *J. School Health* 40:168–172.

Hunt, J.M. 1979. Psychological development: early experience. In M.R. Rosenzweig and L.W. Porter (Eds.): *Annual Reviews in Psychology.* Palo Alto, California: Annual Reviews, 30:103–143.

Kearsley, R.B. 1979. Iatrogenic retardation: a syndrome of learned incompetence. In R.B. Kearsley and I.E. Sigel (Eds.): *Infants at Risk: Assessment of Cognitive Functioning.* Hillsdale, New Jersey: Lawrence Erlbaum Associates, pp. 153–180.

Kinch, R.A. and Kruger, E. 1970. Some sociomedical aspects on the adolescent pregnancy. *Int. J. Gynecol. Obstet.* 8:480.

Kubie, L.A. 1959. Are we educating for maturity? *Natl. Ed. Assoc. J.* 48:58–63.
Lipsitz, J. 1977. *Growing up Forgotten.* Lexington, Massachusetts: Lexington Books.
Marmet, L. 1977. School setting model. In D.J. Bogue (Ed.): *Adolescent Fertility: The Proceedings of an International Conference.* Chicago, Illinois: Community and Family Study Center, University of Chicago.
Morris, L.A. (Ed.). 1977. *Education for Parenthood: A Program, Curriculum, and Evaluation Guide.* Washington, DC: DHEW Publication No. (OHDS) 77-30125.
Osofsky, H.J. and Osofsky, J.D. 1970. Adolescents as mothers; results of a program for low-income pregnant teenagers with some emphasis upon infants' development. *Am. J. Orthopsychiatry* 40:825–834.
Roche, A.F. 1979. Secular trends in human growth, maturation, and development. *Mono. Soc. Res. Child Dev.* 44(3–4).
Sameroff, A.J. 1979. The etiology of cognitive competence: a systems perspective. In R.B. Kearsley and I.E. Sigel (Eds.): *Infants at Risk: Assessment of Cognitive Functioning.* Hillsdale, New Jersey: Lawrence Erlbaum Associates, pp. 115–152.
Sanchez, P.B. 1977. Hot line model. In D.J. Bogue (Ed.): *Adolescent Fertility: The Proceedings of an International Conference.* Chicago, Illinois: Community and Family Study Center, University of Chicago.
Schachter, F.F. 1979. *Everyday Mother Talk to Toddlers: Early Intervention.* New York: Academic Press.
Smith, P.B., Wait, R.B., Mumford, D.M., Nenney, S.W. and Hollins, B.T. 1978. The medical impact of an antepartum program for pregnant adolescents: a statistical analysis. *Am. J. Publ. Health* 68:169–172.
Smith, P.B., Mumford, D.M. and Hamner, E. 1975. Hotline for teenage mothers. *Am. J. Nurs.* 75:1504.
Stine, O.C. and Kelley, E.B. 1970. Evaluation of a school for young mothers: The frequency of prematurity among infants born to mothers under 17 years of age according to the mother's attendance of a special school during pregnancy. *Pediatrics* 46:581–587.
Sugar, M. (Ed.). 1980. *Responding to Adolescent Needs.* New York: Spectrum Publications.
van Doorninck, W.J., Dawson, P., Butterfield, P.M. and Alexander, H.I. 1980. *Parent-Infant Support Through Lay Health Visitors: The Parent Infant Project 1977-1979.* Final Report, Research Grant No. MC-R-080398-03-0, submitted to Maternal and Child Health Service, Bureau of Community Health Service, National Institute of Health Department of Health, Education and Welfare.
von Hippel, C. and Cohen, K.C. 1976. *Summary of Evaluation Findings, Year Two.* Newton, Massachusetts: Education Development Center.
Washington, V.E. 1975. Models of comprehensive service—special school based. *J. School Health* 45:274–277.
Werner, E.E. 1980. Environmental interaction in minimal brain dysfunctions. In H.E. Rie and E.D. Rie (Eds.): *Handbook of Minimal Brain Dysfunction: A Critical View.* New York: John Wiley & Sons, pp. 210–231.
Werner, E.E. and Smith, R.S. 1979. *Vulnerable, But Invincible: A Longitudinal Study of Resilient Children and Youth.* Final report submitted to the Foundation for Child Development, September 30, 1979.

Werner, E.E. and Smith, R.S. 1977. *Kauai's Children Come of Age.* Honolulu, Hawaii: University Press of Hawaii.

Werner, E.E., Bierman, J.M. and French, F.E. 1971. *The Children of Kauai.* Honolulu, Hawaii: University Press of Hawaii.

Wertheim, E.S. 1975. Person-environment interaction: the epigenesis of autonomy and competence. *Br. J. Med. Psychol.* 48:18-8, 95–111, 237–256, 391–402.

Wiegerink, R. and Parrish, V. 1975. A parent implemented preschool program. In D.L. Lillie and P.L. Trohanis (Eds.): *Training Parents to Teach.* New York: Walker & Company.

Zabin, L.S., Kantner, J.F. and Zelnik, M. 1979. The risk of adolescent pregnancy in the first months of intercourse. *Fam. Plann. Perspect.* 11:215.

Zelazo, P.R. 1979. Reactivity to perceptual-cognitive events: application for infant assessment. In R.B. Kearsley and I.E. Sigel (Eds.): *Infants at Risk: Assessment of Cognitive Functioning.* Hillsdale, New Jersey: Lawrence Erlbaum Associates.

Zigler, E. and Valentine, J. (Eds.). 1979. *Project Head Start: A Legacy of the War on Poverty.* New York: The Free Press.

10

Reproductive Health Care for Teens

PEGGY B. SMITH

INTRODUCTION

In response to the growing concern over the consequences of adolescent pregnancy, several models of programmatic intervention have moved beyond remedial levels of service delivery involving the already pregnant adolescent to those providing pregnancy prevention through adolescent reproductive health services. The need for such programs is documented not only by the annual estimate of 1,000,000 pregnant adolescents, but also by the estimate that 50 percent of the four million females aged 15 to 19 years of age are in need of family planning services because of their sexual activity (Tyrer and Josimovich, 1977).

The pregnancy prevention approach, once completely blocked by community resistance (Gordon, 1974), now appears to have gained momentum. This impetus has been augmented by the fact that legislatures and courts continue to affirm the right of young people to seek health care, which includes contraceptive service (Paul et al, 1976). In keeping with the effect of such change, general community attitudes concerning adolescent sexuality seem to have mellowed. A growing national public approval for making contraceptive services available to teenagers keeps the public in step with the courts or vice versa (Gallup, 1978). These trends are not without resistance. Some branches of the medical profession still are reluctant to provide family planning services to minors (Minkler, 1971). However, the official position of both the Academy of Pediatrics and the American College of Obstetrics and Gynecology endorses the preventive approach.

This chapter provides substantive information on the conceptualization, development, implementation, and evaluation of such health care service systems. It focuses on the characteristics of teen programs and teen users, including the adolescent male, and addresses the role of the community in the development of pregnancy prevention programs, especially as it relates to service acceptance. Unless otherwise indicated, the discussion is primarily of the never-pregnant girl and her partner. It is hoped that such information will lead to a better understanding of the ways in which reproductive services can be more effectively provided to adolescents.

COITUS DURING ADOLESCENCE

Despite the notoriety assigned to prevalence of intercourse among adolescents, recent research has confirmed the little publicized fact that the majority of sexually active teens are normal (Lipsitz, 1980) and make the transition from childhood to adulthood relatively unscathed. The evidence of normalcy among this age group is important for its casts teen sexuality as just one component in adolescent development; it is a task to be accomplished rather than pathology to be overcome. Mitchell (1976) corroborated this perception by stating that the need for intimacy is central in adolescent development and influences all adolescent patterns and habits, especially those related to close friendships and romantic interests. Sexual manifestations of this need are usually controlled and conditioned by a variety of social, moral, and ethical constraints which vary among cultural, racial, and social groups.

Sexual activity among adolescents, however, has not always been regarded as normal. Until recently, the tacit assumption was that teenagers were either asexual or that they sublimated all sexual urges until adulthood. Such thinking was possibly facilitated by earlier research (Oliven, 1965) which suggested that adolescents who initiated sexual activity or became pregnant suffered from defects in ego strength and had deep-seated emotional problems. Recent research has reassessed such assumptions and generally suggests that pregnancy in this age group is probably the result of misperception of risk (Zabin et al, 1979) and poor contraceptive utilization (Kantner and Zelnik, 1972), rather than a sign of significant emotional problems.

While the total spectrum of adolescent sexuality has been published elsewhere (Sorenson, 1973; Hass, 1979), coital behavior among adolescents is of interest to those professionals who provide preventive reproductive services. Specifics of intercourse among minors can provide insight into optimal timing of the provision of sex education and contraceptive services, so that proper information and services will be available before pregnancy occurs. The limitations, however, of any discussion of adolescent sexual behavior should first be mentioned. Although patient profiles are available, little is known about why certain women become sexually active at an early age where others defer relations until a more mature time. The selective process is a complex one depending on such factors as dating opportunity, social control, social expectations, and religious influences (Furstenberg, 1976). Profiles of sexually active patients are mentioned later in this chapter, but the underlying motivational factors of that behavior are still conjectural.

The existing data on adolescent intercourse (albeit incomplete) indicate significant behavioral trends in this age group with interrelationships between race, sex, age, and contraceptive usage. Age of first intercourse among teens appears to be declining, and the prevalence of sexual activity appears to be increasing. Estimates made in the 1970s cited that one fourth of white males and females were sexually experienced by age 15 or 16. For blacks, the figure for coitus is estimated at 90 percent for males and 50 percent for females, respectively (Kantner and Zelnik, 1972; Vener and Stewart, 1974; Jessor and Jessor, 1975). More recent research (Zelnik and Kantner, 1978) pointed out that from 1971 to 1976, initiation of premarital intercourse among never-married teens 15 to 19 years of age had increased 41 percent for whites and 19 percent for blacks. One explanation of this rising prevalence is that sexual activity is occurring at younger ages. However, statistical data seem to indicate that early coitus is only partly the answer. The initiation of coital experience has increased in every age category.

Early start of intercourse also seems to be related to effective use of contraception. Cutright (1972) pointed out that the later a female commences sexual activity, the more likely she is to use contraception at the same age. It is noteworthy that only 30 percent of all sexually active females aged 15 used contraception at last intercourse, and that among the sometime users only about 20 percent did so. The fact that a teen is 18 does not, however, guarantee that she will use birth control. Cutright further noted that 50 percent of sexually active teens, including girls 18 years of age, did not use contraception the last time they had intercourse. Recent studies on effective contraception utilization and age of initiation of sexual activity (Zabin et al, 1979) reconfirmed that the very young teen has the greatest risk. Age of first intercourse appears to have a strong effect on the risk of conception. Girls who initiate sexual activity at the youngest ages are at the greatest risk of pregnancy in the early months of exposure, because contraceptive use is greater among girls who initiate sexual activity at a later age. In other words, late starters have a lower risk of conception than do the youngest starters because of the differential use of contraception.

Risk is diminished for girls using medical methods of contraception (pill, intrauterine device; sterilization) as opposed to nonmedical methods including the condom, diaphragm, rhythm, foam, withdrawal, and douche. Regularity of use is an important determinant of risk. Zabin and associates (1979) showed that a higher proportion of black girls conceive largely because of the longer duration of exposure to risk of conception and not due to any greater risk per month exposed. In their study the mean duration of sexual activity of black adolescents aged 18 to 19 was 34 months compared with only 20 months among white girls. Settlage and associates (1973) corroborated timing and racial differential in that the blacks began sexual intercourse at younger ages. However, Settlage and associates found that blacks are more likely than whites to ask for contraception early in their sexual behavior. Mexican-Americans on the other hand, are not likely to use contraception before initiating sexual activity, and fewer have ever used any form of birth control, even though as a group they became sexually active later. The Settlage group further identified economic variables in contraceptive use in that girls from families of lowest income are more likely to delay the longest in asking for birth control after starting coitus.

Of special interest to reproductive health care providers is the number of sexual partners. Risks associated with sexually transmitted diseases, pelvic inflammatory disease, and cancer (Mumford and McCormick, 1980) have been linked to serial sexual contact. Research has demonstrated that while some increase has occurred from 1971 to 1976 in the number of partners, sexually active adolescents usually do not have multiple consorts. Cutright (1972) found that among sexually active teens, there appears to be little promiscuity since in the previous month 90 percent had only one partner. The opportunity for a high degree of promiscuity over the short run does not exist.

The relationships between age, race, and number of partners are subtle. For blacks, there appears to be no relationship between age and number of partners, whereas for the whites there is a slight tendency for the number of partners to increase with age. Given the difference in relationship between age and number of partner for two otherwise essentially similar racial groups, whites appear, if anything, to be somewhat less faithful than blacks. Cutright (1972) suggested that this apparent difference may be due to factors other than race or to the fact that blacks on the average are sexually active for a longer time. However, approximately 40 percent of both races, taking all ages together, have had more than one partner. For each race there is an inverse relationship between age and the proportion of having only one partner, with the relationship being somewhat stronger for whites than blacks. Cutright suggested that while proportionately more blacks than whites have intercourse, it is the whites who have sex more frequently and are more promiscuous.

A brief perusal of the literature indicates a constellation of excuses for nonutilization of birth control that are independent of chronologic age or racial breakdown. The most frequently cited reasons given by sexually active teens were that they generally did not think they could become pregnant or that they disbelieved in their reproductive capability (Zackler and Brandstandt, 1975; Kantner and Zelnik, 1972; Sorenson, 1973). Cutright (1972) indicated that blacks were inclined to feel that they were infertile, whereas whites were more inclined to rely on the menstrual cycle for protection.

Another related reason in contraceptive nonuse or misuse involves ignorance and misinformation (Essler, 1978). Minkowsky and associates (1974) found striking ignorance concerning basic anatomy and sexuality which corroborates previously cited research; when questioned, most teens indicated their belief that mid-cycle was the best time to have unprotected intercourse.

Psychological factors have also been identified as significant in the non-utilization of birth control. Tyrer and Josimovich (1977) cited a variety of psychological considerations associated with contraception. In the developing teenager's self-concept of sexual identity there is often little understanding of the consequences of intercourse. Teenagers frequently have ambivalence and guilt about sexual activity, along with anxiety and inner conflict about contraceptive responsibility. In her study of abortion and the decision not to contracept, Luker (1975) found that in some cases females perceived the risks of pregnancy more positively than the benefits of contraception. This phenomenon is especially true for teens. Such psychological factors involving teens are conditioned by the total life situation, stage of development, and related life-styles of involved adolescents, and suggest that education by itself will probably make little impact on their contraceptive practices. It should be pointed out that most teens do not engage in intercourse for the purpose of becoming pregnant. Many see sex as necessary for the social rewards of dating (Klein, 1978), meaning that intercourse is the price a teen girl must pay if she is to be popular. But as mentioned earlier, there are factors often beyond the girl's control which do not facilitate the inclusion of contraception in this social arena.

REPRODUCTIVE CLINIC FORMAT AND SERVICES

In response to this growing body of data documenting the health and sexual needs of teens, a variety of health care delivery models has been developed. The types of services provided in these models may reflect the general orientation of the provider, the needs of the adult community, or the requirements of the teen population. One of the first types of health clinics designed for teens was traditional, with a format similar to the total health care model for adults offering services by medical or pediatric professionals. Such medical efforts emphasized general health screening and treatment and were often free-standing (usually in poverty areas) or school-based. The treated conditions in these programs often reflect health problems prevalent in the adult population, such as hypertension, dental caries, skin disorders, and poor nutrition.

In a series of school-based health assessments of adolescents, Rogers and Reese (1965) found that physical appraisals of so-called healthy students revealed a high prevalence of visual, dental, and skin conditions. Further exploration of utilization patterns manifested by those adolescents who frequented the clinic for physical complaints found that these teens were also considered to have a higher frequency of social and emotional problems than their classmates. Unfortunately, the serial investigations of Rogers and Reese provide little insight into the sexual investigations or reproductive conditions of minors since genital examinations and questions concerning sexuality or reproduction were not permitted. Such regulations precluded screening for sexually transmitted diseases as well.

General medical programs for adolescents were also established in inner-city clinics. While such locations still utilized the traditional adult medical formats, a more liberal orientation to sexual health could be fostered.

From assessment in school-based clinics, the primary health problems identified by Brunswick and Josephson (1972) were dental, respiratory, and nutritional. Reproductive concerns such as menstrual disorders, pregnancy, or genital tract disorders were found in less than four percent of the girls interviewed. The findings from (Salisbury and Berg, 1969; Eisner et al, 1966) programs associated with summer work or job corps applicants are similar to those of school and clinic-based programs, with dental disease, hypertension, and heart disease being the most prevalent major problems. No attempts to screen, treat, or discuss reproductive concerns or conditions were reported from these sources.

From the brief review of general health clinics for adolescents, it appears that traditional health programs do not provide (or perhaps avoid) any in-depth assessment and delivery of reproductive services to their teen clients. Even though the deletion of reproductive services in settings such as schools or job screening programs is understandable, the prevalence of sexually related concerns (including venereal disease) in this age group necessitates the inclusion of this component into adolescent medical services. The recent proliferation of clinics of this type seems to support this assumption. The Alan Guttmacher Institute (1976) estimated that in 1975, 1,175,000 teenagers attended reproductive or contraceptive programs at 5,272 locations; the teenage caseload represented 30 percent of the 3.9 million family planning patients reported by organized United States projects.

The delivery of reproductive health care seems to be especially suited to specialty or family planning clinics. A popular format which facilitates this service delivery is the establishment of special reproductive clinics with staff especially selected to meet the needs of sexually active teens. Grouping teens together maximizes the delivery of confidential services since they won't be sitting in the clinic with older women whom they may know. House and Goldsmith (1972) pointed out that younger girls are especially apt to be quite nervous about their first pelvic exam and need more support. Special clinics can also provide flexible scheduling, including evening and Saturday hours, to accommodate the adolescent's school programs. Sex education, contraceptive information and materials, pregnancy and venereal disease testing, and counseling for abortion or prenatal care (Goldsmith et al, 1972) are also easily provided in special teen clinics. To date, approximately one third of teenage family planning or reproductive health services are provided in this manner (Coughlin and Perales, 1978).

Not all health care providers choose to reach teens through the separate clinic approach since some professionals feel that sexually active adolescents should be treated and considered as adults. Staffing problems and logistic constraints preclude the establishment of separate clinics for others. To maximize teen utilization for both models, four strategies have been suggested by Brann and associates (1979): the intense one on one, the provision of everything at one site approach, the broadcast approach, and the standard outreach combined with easy access to abortion approach. The inclusion of one or more of these strategies appears to enhance program effectiveness. Specific examples of some of these strategies are discussed in the evaluation section of this chapter.

SERVICE CRITERIA

A variety of service criteria can be identified as maximizing adolescent use of reproductive or family planning clinics and which are applicable in separate and integrated clinics. Poole (1976) found that adolescents specifically wanted education concerning sex and drugs, venereal disease and contraception, pregnancy testing, counseling and alternatives to handling pregnancy, as well as information concerning normal growth and development. These findings are compatible with those of earlier traditional health care models (Brunswick and Josephson, 1972; Salisbury and Berg, 1969) in which adolescents expressed the need to know whether or not they were normal.

House and Goldsmith (1972) identified three primary elements which were central to the success of family planning facilities for teens. These were convenience, staff, and decor. They stipulated that the optimal setting had to have easy accessibility by public transportation or walking and a location where teens could go without embarassing encounters with adults. Minkowski and associates (1974) indicated that staffing attitudes and general climate should convince adolescents that they are important and are treated with respect and dignity. Decor, on the other hand, does not seem to be an important concern. The American College of Obstetrics and Gynecology (1979) emphasized the importance of the availability of contraception without parental consent and without charge.

The Urban and Rural Systems Associate study (URSA, 1976) identified types of criteria in the priorities and relationships of the various services requested by adolescents. The first group consisted of threshold conditions which must be met in order for teens to attend the clinic and included clinic availability, a guarantee of confidentiality and anonymity, and affordability. Once these three conditions were met, the secondary factors that influenced teens to make an initial visit were location, easy transportation, convenience of clinic hours, length of appointment visit, and ease of admission. Less important to most teenagers surveyed were the sex, age, and dress of the clinician or staff member, staff professional qualifications, teen-oriented decor, and exclusively teen clinic sessions.

The URSA study (1976) also noted barriers that contributed to the clinics' lack of success in reaching teens. These including restrictive (or perceived) state legislation which limit younger teens' access to birth control without parental consent, federal trends toward cutting back funds and consequent increased reliance by clinics on patient fees and third party payments, and federal funding policies that impose limits on providing services. The lack of community acceptance of the services or such a perception by clinic staff often provided a psychological barrier to service delivery to minors. Many clinic staff members indicated that they felt a lack of support for their services in general and a need to keep a low profile from the media in order to avoid potential community backlash.

Although certain basic services are important in the delivery of reproductive health care to teens, the level of implementation varies from provider to provider. A federally sponsored national survey (Coughlin and Perales, 1978) that attempted to ascertain the level of actual teen health services in a variety of settings found that, in general, teen planning clinics were housed in orderly, clean, and physically attractive surroundings, although in some facilities, especially in the south, clinic sites were somewhat small and austere. Services were generally accessible, but transportation was a problem in the rural areas. Most of the services were affordable, and teenagers were rarely turned away from family planning services because of the inability to pay. The majority of the adolescent clients became aware of the clinic through informal referral by friends and acquaintances.

However, major threshold problems (as defined by URSA) were lack of confidentiality and preappointment waiting periods which still existed as obstacles to greater attendance. In almost half of the providers, teenagers expressed strong fears of parental knowledge of their sexual activity or clinic involvement. Almost three fourths of the providers indicated that teenagers had to wait anywhere from several days to several weeks, and the time in the clinic was anywhere from two to four hours. Male involvement was also seen as a problem in the clinic, as were the referral systems and the limited counseling available. A major barrier to providing information services for teens to control their own fertility was a negative community attitude, indicating the indispensable need to mobilize community action.

CLINIC PUBLICITY

Clinic publicity is an important variable that facilitates teen patient initiation and continuation in reproductive health care. Publicity concerning clinic functions helps to create general awareness of the need for family planning and the need to inform teens of the availability of services. The accomplishment of these two objectives is a delicate process. To be effective, one must be educated on the target population's needs without stimulating the ire of ultraconservative groups which may not as yet perceive the need for such reproductive health care activities. A variety of techniques is available to perform this task. The media probably constitute the most potent communicator with the adolescent age group. The radio is an especially effective tool since music seems to be an integral part of the adolescent's lifestyle and possesses a certain flexibility which the television lacks; radio campaigns (Department of Health, Education, and Welfare [DHEW], 1979), using rock stars and movie celebrities, may enhance this already powerful communicator.

Brochures and pamphlets may also provide publicity especially if they are at the language level of and meet the informational needs of the users. The inclusion of city and building maps on the back of brochures can also provide a sense of security for the patient who makes it to the front door. Brochures suitable for mailing in a regular letter size envelope provide a discreet cover for those individuals who would like to receive the information privately. Wallet-sized cards may also provide an effective way to pass pertinent information among the target age groups.

Probably the most powerful recruitment publicity for teen services is word of mouth. In a recent teen clinic assessment (Nenney and Smith, 1983), the most frequently cited referral source by sexually active never-pregnant adolescents was a close friend or family acquaintance. Personal contact with health care providers who work with the adolescents in the schools is another vehicle for clinic publicity. School nurses can provide an invaluable educational liaison and referral source for high-risk patients for specific counseling and/or family planning needs. In addition, nurses can help to organize trips to reproductive clinical facilities in which programs can be presented under the auspices of the learning experience of a field trip.

The context in which the clinic is described is probably more important than publicity sources. Although healthy sexual performance and functioning are admirable, clinics that provide reproductive services for sexually active adolescents should not primarily present themselves as "methods courses." Similarly, the remediation of sexual dysfunction (as by Masters and Johnson) should be avoided. Although such goals are admirable in the larger scheme of things, they are political suicide to preventive pregnancy programs for adolescents.

COMMUNITY AND TEEN REPRODUCTIVE HEALTH

Positive community rapport is essential to successful implementation and delivery of reproductive health services to adolescents; in its absence, a clinic's effort to reach and serve the adolescent patient will be significantly crippled. Community acceptance can be a very powerful force for the good. Past efforts of interested community members in fields such as mental retardation and birth defects illustrate the value of the grassroots movement in bringing about change in previously unchangeable or controversial areas. In most communities there is little quarrel with data documenting the prevalence of venereal disease and unwanted pregnancies. Parents are appalled by the evidence of youthful sexuality. However, such data are quickly attributed to other populations in the community with whom little mutuality exists.

Denial of the sexuality of one's own children may provide a defense mechanism for parents who may be psychologically overwhelmed by the possibility that their own children are sexually active. Furstenberg (1976) found that most mothers preferred to believe that their daughters were not having sexual relations, enabling them to put off any discussion of the matter until the need arose. Sexual activity for this group not only violated community sexual mores, but catapulted mothers into discussions for whch they were ill prepared and poorly informed. Thus, denial of the total sexual phenomenon was the alternative most often chosen. Minkowski and associates (1974) suggested that the underlying motivation for this community posture may run the gamut from genuine concern for premature sexual involvement and the potential impact upon physical and emotional health to fear of the real or imagined consequences. This kind of denial on the part of the community middle class may not always be self-serving. In the past, statistics gathered from studies of teen pregnancy were usually retrieved from public or charity clinics which served predominantly the poor or minority groups. Teen records from the private clinics, on the other hand, working with middle or upper class adolescents who had pregnancies were not, and are not, as accessible. Thus, when public health data are retrieved and interpretations extracted, the behavior of a large segment of nonpoor teenagers is not represented in the data base. Community members therefore really do not have substantive data or information on their own children but only on the children of the poor.

Thus, one of the first steps in enlisting community support should be to convince all segments of the community that adolescent sexuality is an equally distributed community phenomenon. While national data are impressive, local statistics reflecting the current status of adolescent pregnancy, abortion, and sexually transmitted disease may in the long run eliminate community denial.

Once reproductive health professionals convince the local community of the existing need, programs should continue to enlist community involvement by including both the adolescent consumer and the adult community. Continuing involvement can take a variety of forms. Utilization of such interested parties as volunteers can simultaneously maximize clinical services, minimize overhead, and provide informal community advocacy. Community and clinic teaching are options for those who want to be actively involved. Other community members' interests can be channeled toward administrative activities such as the assemblage of educational material, coordination of information in a newsletter format, or acquisition or recycling of objects for clinic use. As "private citizens," such persons can also enlighten others to the goal that services provide. When political or controversial issues threaten such service provision, project volunteers can speak in behalf of rendered services. Teen volunteers can provide especially valuable services as potential users. Participation by teens in program planning can be a sensitive source of information and policy development concerning the special needs of target groups.

Community involvement should not be undertaken without caution. Although volunteers, especially teens, have been credited with increasing patient participation, confidentiality of patient records may be jeopardized when volunteers are used in teen reproductive health clinics. In addition, teen volunteers and adolescent advisory groups may not provide valid consumer input. Most teenagers who constitute the advisory membership are often chosen in a nonrandom manner and such representation may consist of homogenous populations which lack the entire range of life experience and perspectives.

MALE ROLE IN TEEN REPRODUCTIVE PROGRAMS

The literature on research or service descriptions concerning the contraceptive needs, attitudes, and behavior of adolescent boys is almost nonexistent. The informational and programmatic gap reflects the general state of the art of family planning services for the male population as a whole. There are several reasons for the minimal emphasis on the "male component." Orientation and interest in reproductive health concerns have not been established as a priority item for adolescent males. Brunswick (1971) indicated that girls are considerably more aware of, and concerned about, sex-related matters such as pregnancy, reproduction, and venereal disease than are boys. Boys, on the other hand, are more interested in whether or not they are healthy. Such orientations may ultimately reflect personal attitudinal components which covertly imply that since the consequences of intercourse fall more heavily on the female, the specific behavioral antecedents of coitus such as family planning are primarily female issues.

Culture's inequitable assignment of sex roles also may be partially responsible for male disinterest in reproductive health. Chilman (1978) pointed out that teenage boys are quite casual when it comes to taking responsibility for their sexuality and its consequences, reflecting the way society has treated males from childhood until maturity. In the recent past, the family, school, and community have not expected male sexual responsibility for contraception or teen fatherhood. Predictably, teenage boys who find themselves facing these roles live up to these minimal expectations.

Irresponsible male behavior in the recent past has been supported by the traditional double standard. Miller and Simon (1974) pointed out that unlike females, males were expected to have casual sex with minimal emphasis on the consequences of such actions. This cavalier approach to sexual responsibility appears to have been tacitly supported by female perceptions of reproductive health. In a comprehensive survey of teen recipients of aid (Aid to Families with Dependent Children), Essler (1978) found that the majority of adolescent females felt that most men do not like birth control. Such a belief is especially predominant among low income teens and in Mexican-American ethnic groups. Minkowski and associates (1974) corroborated prevalence of casual male sexual encounters by pointing to the difficulties associated with involving male participation in family planning programs.

This unilateral placement of sexual responsibility is tacitly reinforced by the limited variety of effective male methods of birth control. Coitus interruptus, the condom, and vasectomy are presently the primary male methods available. The condom is the only effective method appropriate for the adolescent male, and its utilization, in the recent past, by this age group may be on the wane. As a result, family planning service delivery systems in the past have developed a strong female orientation by default and have made no extensive effort to attract or involve the male partners in the decision to use contraception. This is corroborated by many facilities that lack male staff members and, in some cases, restrooms for men, in family planning clinics.

The one-sided nonmale orientation, among the general population, however, seems to be gradually changing. The increased interest in vasectomy by men appears to indicate their heightened sense of responsibility for decisions in the area of family planning. The literature indicates that sterilization is now ranked as the most popular method.

Moreover, the rights and responsibilities of putative fathers have recently been substantiated legally. In the Stanley vs. Illinois Decision (1972), the rights of the single father in the area of child custody were given equal protection under the law. This decision was strengthened by the Rothstein vs. Lutheran Social Service Decision (1972), which again guaranteed the rights of the father before the adoption procedures of an illegitimate child could be consummated.

Female coital trends, collected in the late 1960s, also show a gradual attitudinal shift in sexual expectations. Miller and Simon (1974) reported an increase in the incidence of premarital coitus among young women, while male rates have continued to be stable. The approaching attainment of equal sexual experience between the sexes could possibly indicate the beginnings of a trend to equal assignment of responsibility for contraceptive utilization. Unfortunately, trends initiated in the adult population are slow in reaching the adolescent constituency.

As the male's responsibility concerning his contraceptive behavior and his legal right to his progeny (albeit illegitimate) is now becoming apparent, new attention has been focused on various aspects of male behavior related to sexual activity and reproductive health. The Alan Guttmacher Institute (1976) estimated that 65 percent of all teenage men have had intercourse. Applying this proportion to the 10.6 million men aged 15 to 19 years in 1975, the Institute estimated that 6,890,000 teen males were sexually active. The vast majority of their female partners, are, on the average, two years younger than the male (Goldfarb et al, 1977; Zelnik and Kantner, 1978). This age differential is significant for all ethnic groups. Finkel and Finkel (1975) found that the average age of first male sexual activity was 12.8 years. Furstenberg (1976) noted that by age 14, two thirds of the males surveyed were sexually active.

Male contraceptive methods, although considered to be underutilized by the teen population, play a major role in the prevention of pregnancy. In spite of the effectiveness of the intrauterine device and hormonal methods of contraception, research indicates that the condom is the primary contraceptive method for sexually active adolescents (Settlage et al, 1973). Although adolescents complain about the interference with spontaneity and naturalness of coitus, in 44 percent of the cases in which some form of contraception was used, the condom remained the method of choice.

Although somewhere between 40 and 60 percent of sexually active single adolescents of both races depend on the condom (Gobble et al, 1969), and while it is the most frequently listed method used by men, the condom is considered to be underused and its popularity has actually declined. Between 1965 and 1975, condom use fell off for all groups (Westoff, 1976). Such contraceptive patterns among teens are disturbing, since the condom has been cited as especially suitable to the adolescent population that engages in sporadic or occasional sex. Moreover, since the 15- to 25-year-old age group contributes 65 percent of the cases of venereal disease, the condom offers potential health maintenance benefits (Redford et al, 1974). Additional psychological factors have the potential to enhance condom utilization. The possession of contraceptives by girls not only belies their romantic belief in the spontaneity of sex but may be found by their parents as incriminating evidence of their daughters' sexual activity. Young women carrying contraceptives may also be regarded as signaling their sexual availability. Society does not castigate the male so much as the female for premarital sex and the possession of condoms (Ewing and Visco, 1978).

In spite of these perceived advantages, why are adolescents unable to utilize the condom effectively on a greater scale? A variety of reasons has been suggested, and they run the gamut of nonaggressive marketing to the dimunition of sensual pleasure. Harvey (1973) suggested that widespread use of the condom has been inhibited because of its past association with venereal disease prevention and prostitution. Rumel and associates (1971) stated that the pharmacist needs to be more aggressive in projecting a positive image for the condom, including easier accessibility. It appears that having to ask for the condom, especially on the part of teen males, is a real deterrent to effective utilization. This may explain why vending machines were the preferred place of purchase (Gilbert and Matthews, 1974).

Adolescent male utilization of contraception can be enhanced or inhibited by the relationships with the female partner. Ewing and Visco (1978) believed that good communication between partners is an extension for role-sharing behavior, which includes birth control. Luker (1975) on the other hand, suggested that in casual sexual relationships the teen male concern for the protection of the female partner may be negated by the belief that female methods are readily available.

Although the literature documents the need for reproductive health services for adolescent males, only two types of service providers are readily apparent in the literature. The condom appears to be the most significant method of choice. Attempts have been made to distribute free condoms to adolescent boys through barber shops, pool halls, grocery stores, and restaurants. Arnold and Cogswell's (1971) results with this approach indicated that if boys are given a chance, they will become increasingly more willing to share in the family planning responsibilities (Gobble et al, 1969).

The rap session is another approach designed to reach the adolescent male. Such sessions provide information on contraception, decision making, human sexuality, and moral issues in sexual behavior. Male involvement in mixed counseling groups appears to have an especially positive effect with improved quality of the sessions, since its permits dialogue between the sexes (House and Goldsmith, 1972). Such a format, however, has not been widely accepted or implemented.

While the importance of adolescent male involvement in reproductive health is widely endorsed by providers (Chilman, 1978), limited service options indicate that professionals probably know less about how to provide services to the male adolescent than to any other male age group (Jekel, 1975). Family planning demographic information corroborates this lack of expertise by indicating that active male participation is minimal. Nenney and Smith (1983) found that despite extensive outreach and publicity techniques, male participation was marginal. For those male teens who actively participated, attendance involved participation for noncontraceptive reasons. However, a group of males informally observed as nonregistered friends of attending girls in the teen clinic were possibly involved in a passive family planning role. Approximately 30 percent of previously pregnant girls coming in for postpartum exams were accompanied by a male partner, but the reason for such companionship is often unclear. Perhaps such couples had a more mature approach to birth control as a joint responsibility, or the girl needed an on-site babysitter or clinic transportation, or the male actually provided moral support for contraceptive compliance. These observations suggest, however, that a greater effort might enlist formal male participation.

A data pool that may provide insight into teen male reproductive health is research on unwed teen fathers. Klerman (1975) found that when fathers were involved during the pregnancy, a marriage resulted which in turn led to another early pregnancy. Such a result obviously may be counterproductive to the ultimate goal of reproductive health programs for teens.

Furstenberg (1976) observed that at the one-year follow-up, 20 percent of the mothers had lost touch with their partners, which increased to 37 percent at the five-year follow-up. Therefore, involvement of the father may bind the couple into a marital contract that is short-lived, with 'high probability of failure," and which will result in greater parity for the adolescent mother.

It appears, therefore, that a significant male involvement in reproductive health care is greatly needed and that innovative techniques hold some potential. Some authors (Essler, 1978) suggested that considerable educational efforts need to be directed at males, particularly younger ones, in order to bring home to them the advantages of birth control and the disadvantages of having their girlfriends become pregnant. Such an approach must proceed in a sensitve way. Educational attempts in the past have emphasized the negative aspects of male participation in intercourse. Phrases such as "would you be more careful if it were you that got pregnant," while widely appealing to females, may stimulate escape-avoidance behavior in the adolescent male rather than motivate responsibility for his sexual activity.

EVALUATION OF FAMILY PLANNING PROGRAMS FOR TEENS

Since growing public concern has brought about an increase in federal interest and subsequent fundings, a variety of model programs has been developed which address the sexual development and behavior of adolescents. They use a wide variety of service models and include sex education courses, broad-casting strategies, multi-purpose centers, counseling for young people and/or parents, contraceptive and abortion services, treatment for venereal disease, special programs for unwed parents and their children, and public assistance. It therefore would be very useful to have some idea of the relative effectiveness of these models. Brann and associates (1979) pointed out that this information would be extremely helpful, so that programs to prevent unintended child-bearing by teenagers could be compared with programs to ameliorate the adverse consequences of motherhood for teens. At this time such information, on a comprehensive basis, does not exist.

Several attempts were made in the 1970s to provide such substantive infor-mation on a national and a selected local basis. These evaluations provided infor-mation on reaching the adolescent as well as evaluation of outcome objectives of specific programs. The largest circulated study to date (Alan Guttmacher Insti-tute, 1976), in which contraceptive services for adolescents were assessed by county and state for the year 1975, indicated that since 1969 the estimated number of teenage patients had in fact increased in the United States from 214,000 to almost 1.2 million, and the proportion of total caseload represented by adolescents aged 15 to 19 years has grown from 20 to 30 percent. This study, which hypothesized that one measure of effectiveness could be determined by the availability of service, reported that there were 592 counties in 1975 that had no family planning services for adolescents; with a few exceptions, the same counties had no family planning services at all. Although many of these counties were rural and had relatively small numbers of adolescents at risk, each of 153 counties had 300 or more adolescents at risk, a number which was judged suffi-cient to warrant the consideration of family planning services. An interesting correlation with the percentage of teenagers served is the percentage of all low and marginal income women in need that are served. The Alan Guttmacher Insti-tute found that the majority of countries that are more effective in serving teenagers are also more effective in serving low and marginally income women. This suggests that a key independent variable would be the limited income of adolescents in determining their choice of a public clinic.

The Alan Guttmacher Institute also demonstrated a relationship between the variety of agencies in the community and the improved effectiveness in reaching the teen. Through their analysis, the proportion of adolescents at risk by organized programs seems to vary directly with a number of types and pro-vider agencies in the county: 24 percent of the teen need was served in single agency counties, 32 percent of the teen need in two agency counties, 34 per-cent of the teen need in three agency counties, and 38 percent of the need in counties with all types of providers, thus documenting the rationale for having variance in delivery format to the adolescent.

Once the adolescent has been reached and has been provided with accessible services, how well are the individual objectives of those services met? The most difficult question to be answered involves the documentation of programmatic effect on fertility, knowledge, or behavioral outcome. Through an onsite assessment of a variety of programs for teenagers around the country, Brann and associates (1979) located and documented programs as utilizing different models which actualized change in outcome objectives. A clinic in St. Paul, Minnesota, organized through a Maternal and Infant Care project, which established a goal of reducing birth rates in the student population, was able to show the following results: the percentage of mothers dropping out of school subsequent to delivery decreased from 45 to less than 10 percent; all continuing young mothers accepted contraception and there have been no repeat pregnancies; the staff is aware of no accidental pregnancies among this age group; the fertility rate decreased from 79 per 1,000 in 1972 and 1973 to 35 per 1,000 in 1975 and 1976. The conclusion drawn was that the program contributed to the decrease in birth rate.

Humboldt County, California has a successful family life education program with quantifiable results. A 20-month follow-up of 50 participants with documented sexual activity indicated that not one pregnancy had occurred. Implementers attributed program participation as the significant factor in lowering pregnancy rates (Berg, 1979).

Brann and associates (1979) cited a program sponsored by Planned Parenthood of Maryland in which family planning services, sex education curriculum, and teacher training workshops were conducted. Evaluation in three of the six counties in which the program was implemented indicated that the combined fertility rates for 15 to 19 year olds changed from 84 to 56 births per 1,000 females from 1972 to 1975, a 33 percent drop. In the 15- to 17-year-old age group, usually viewed as a harder age group to reach, the rate decreased from 66 per 1,000 to 42 per 1,000—a 36 percent drop. These are very large changes in a three-year period. Such statistics are cited as preliminary evidence that the programs are working.

Unfortunately, documentation of program effectiveness similar to these evaluation efforts, although critical to the state of the art and continuation of funding, are not widely undertaken. A frequent difficulty in implementing effective evaluation may be due to a general lack of understanding of the concept of evaluation. In the broad sense, a program that attempts to determine how well it is doing without use of clear criteria may be regarded as a valiant though primitive evaluation effort. Measures reflecting percentages of participants, attitude changes, behavior, and compliance all could easily be adapted to programs which serve sexually active teens. Many programs lack stated, defined goals and objectives which can be quantified and measured, without which clearly defined outcome objective measurements cannot be undertaken. When such a process is applied to family planning, the objectives usually focus on birth control and abortion, which are related to the prevention of unwanted births. Such objective outcome is quite important, but long-range design and research based on a proper and reliable methodology are necessary to document that the objective was actually accomplished.

SUMMARY

The development of family planning services for teens comes partially in response to growing public awareness of the prevalence of sexual activity, sexually transmitted disease, and unplanned pregnancy in this age group. Partially, it is in response to the need for sexual and reproductive screening, medical care, and counseling not previously provided by traditional general medical services.

The basic challenges facing such reproductive health programs are multifaceted and not without pitfalls. Staff and administration must have a working knowledge of sexual profiles of minors, understand motivational factors associated with contraceptive utilization, and provide services in a format attractive to a teen clientele. Once services are established, programs must guarantee continued clinic function through ongoing evaluation. Such reproductive clinical functions, however, do not totally address all the issues in reproductive health care for teens. Continuing funding and research is needed to develop more effective ways to evaluate programs and to reach high risk teens, including the very young adolescent and, especially, her male partner. Until these two previously untended groups are reached in a pro-active way, reproductive health care programs for teens and associated service delivery will not maximize their preventive potential.

REFERENCES

Alan Guttmacher Institute. 1976. Contraceptive services for adolescents. *Eleven Million Teenagers.* New York, pp. 1–64.
American College of Obstetrics and Gynecology. 1979. Characteristics of sexually active adolescents. *Adol. Perinatal Health* pp. 1–40.
Arnold, C. B. and Cogswell, B. E. 1971. A condom distribution program for adolescents. *Am. J. Publ. Health* 61(4):739–750.
Berg, P. 1979. *The Effect of a Group Module Program on 50 Women Seeking Family Planning Counseling as Measured by Their Subsequent Pregnancy Rates.* Humboldt-Del Norte County, California: Department of Public Health.

Brann, E. A., Edwards, L., Callicott, T., Story, E. S., Berg, P. A., Mahoney, J. E., Stine, J. L. and Hixson, A. 1979. *Strategies for the Prevention of Pregnancy in Adolescents.* U.S. Department of Health, Education, and Welfare, Public Health Service. Center for Disease Control, Atlanta, Georgia.

Brunswick, A. F. 1971. Adolescent health, sex, and fertility. *Am. J. Publ. Health* 61(4):711-729.

Brunswick, A. F. and Josephson, E. 1972. Adolescent health in Harlem. *Am. J. Publ. Health (Suppl):* 3-60. October.

Chilman, C. S. 1978. *Adolescent Sexuality in a Changing American Society. Social and Psychological Perspectives.* U.S. Department of Health, Education, and Welfare. Public Health Service, National Institute of Health. DHEW Publication No. (NIH) 79-1426.

Coughlin, I. D. J. and Perales, C. A. 1978. *Family Planning and the Teenager, A Service Delivery Assessment.* Report to the Secretary of HEW, New York: November.

Cutright, P. 1972. Illegitimacy in the United States: 1920-1968. The Commission on Population Growth and the American Future. In C. F. Westoff and R. Parke, Jr. (Eds.): *Demographic and Social Aspects of Population Growth.* Vol. I of Commission Research Reports. Washington, DC: Government Printing Office.

Department of Health, Education, and Welfare. National Clearinghouse for Information, 1979. *Using the Media to Approve Family Service Delivery.* November, No. 13.

Eisner, V., Goodlett, C. B. and Driver, M. B. 1966. Health enrollees in neighborhood youth corps. *Pediatrics* 38(1):40-43.

Essler, J. 1978. *Utilization of Family Planning Services by AFDC Recipients in Texas.* A study done for the Texas Department of Human Resources Program Evaluation Division, John H. Winters Building, Austin, Texas.

Ewing, E. and Visco, E. 1978. *Model Programs for Involving Men in Family Planning.* A final report for the Office of Family Planning, Bureau of Community Health Services. Submitted by the National Institute for Community Development, Arlington, Virginia.

Finkel, M. L. and Finkel, D. J. 1975. Sexual and contraceptive knowledge, attitudes and behavior of male adolescents. *Fam. Plann. Perspect.* 7(6):256-260.

Furstenberg, F. F. 1976. *Unplanned Parenthood, The Social Consequences of Teenage Childbearing.* New York: The Free Press.

Gallup, G. 1978. Epidemic of teen pregnancies: growing number of Americans favor discussion of sex in the classroom. *The Gallup Poll.* Princeton, New Jersey: News Release, January 23.

Gilbert, R. and Matthews, V. G. 1974. Young male's attitudes toward condom use. In M. Redford, G. Duncan, and D. Prager (Eds.): *The Condom: Increasing Utilization in the U.S.* San Francisco: San Francisco Press, pp. 164-172.

Gobble, F. L., Clark, E. V., Cochran, C. M. and Lock, F. R. 1969. A nonmedical approach to fertility reduction—an experimental contraceptive service unit. *Obstet. Gynecol.* 34(6):888-891.

Goldfarb, J. L., Mumford, D. M., Schum, D. A., Smith, P. B., Flowers, C. and Schum, C. 1977. An attempt to detect "pregnancy susceptibility" in indigent adolescent girls. *J. Youth Adol.* 6(2):127-144.

Goldsmith, S., Gabrielson, M. O., Gabrielson, I., Matthews, V. and Potts, L. 1972. Teenagers, sex and contraception. *Fam. Plann. Perspect.* 4(1):32–38.

Gordon, S. 1974. Why sex education belongs in the home. *The PTA Magazine.* February, pp. 15–17.

Harvey, P. D. 1973. Marketing birth control. In M. McMillan (Ed.): *Using Commercial Resources in Family Planning Communication Programs: The International Experience.* Honolulu: University Press of Hawaii, pp. 31–33.

Hass, A. 1979. *Teenage Sexuality: A Survey of Teenage Sexual Behavior.* New York: MacMillan.

House, E. A. and Goldsmith, S. 1972. Planned parenthood services for the young teenager. *Fam. Plann. Perspect.* 4(2):27–31.

Jekel, J. F. 1975. Appraising programs for school-age parents. *J. School Health* 45:296–300.

Jessor, S. and Jessor, R. 1975. Transition from virginity to nonvirginity among youth: a social-psychological study over time. *Dev. Psychol.* 11(4):473–484.

Kantner, J. F. and Zelnik, M. 1972. Sexual experiences of young unmarried women in the U.S. *Fam. Plann. Perspect.* 4:9–17.

Klein, L. 1978. Antecedents of teenage pregnancy. *Clin. Obstet. Gynecol.* 2(4):1151–1160.

Klerman, L. V. 1975. Adolescent pregnancy, the need for new policies and new programs. *J. School Health* 45:263–267.

Lipsitz, J. S. 1980. Adolescent psychosexual development. In P. B. Smith and D. Mumford (Eds.): *Adolescent Pregnancy: Perspectives for the Health Professional.* Boston: G. K. Hall.

Luker, K. 1975. *Taking Chances: Abortion and the Decision Not to Contracept.* National Institute for Community Development. Berkley: University of California Press.

Miller, P. Y. and Simon, W. 1974. Adolescent sexual behavior. Context and change. *J. Social Prob.* 22(1):58–76.

Minkler, D. H. 1971. Fertility regulation for teenagers. *Clin. Obstet. Gynecol.* 14:420–431.

Minkowski, W. L., Weiss, R. C., Lawther, L., Shonick, H. and Heidbreder, G. A. 1974. Family planning services for adolescents and young adults. *West. J. Med.* 120:116–123.

Mitchell, J. J. 1976. Adolescent intimacy. *Adolescence* 11(42):275–280.

Mumford, D. M. and McCormick, N. 1980. Venereal disease and the adolescent. In P. B. Smith and D. Mumford (Eds.): *Adolescent Pregnancy: Perspectives for the Health Professional.* Boston: G. K. Hall.

Nenney, S. W. and Smith, P. N. 1983. Teenagers' assessment of reproductive health care services. *Patient Counselling and Health Education* 4(3):152–155.

Oliven, J. F. 1965. *Sexual Hygiene and Pathology, A Manual for the Physician and the Professions.* Philadelphia: J. B. Lippincott.

Paul, E. W., Pilpel, H. R. and Wechsler, N. F. 1976. Pregnancy, teenagers and the law, 1976. *Fam. Plann. Perspect.* 8:16–21.

Poole, C. 1976. Contraception in the adolescent female. *J. School Health* 46(8):253–260.

Redford, M. 1974. Introduction. In M. Redford, G. Duncan, and D. Prager (Eds.): *The Condom: Increasing Utilization in the United States.* San Francisco: San Francisco Press, pp. 15–25.

Rogers, K. D. and Reese, G. 1965. Health studies—presumably normal high school students. *Am. J. Dis. Child.* 109:9–26.

Rothstein v. Lutheran Social Services of Wisconsin and Upper Michigan. 92 S.Ct. 1488, 1972.

Rumel, M. J., Reich, L., Stringfellow, L. and Pian, R. J. 1971. The pharmacist's neglected role. *Fam. Plann. Perspect.* 3(4):80–82.

Salisbury, A. J. and Berg, R. B. 1969. Health defects and need for treatment of adolescents in low income families. *Publ. Health Rep.* 84(8):705–711.

Settlage, D. S. F., Baroff, S. and Cooper, D. 1973. Sexual experience of younger teenage girls seeking contraceptive assistance for the first time. *Fam. Plann. Perspect.* 5(4):233.

Sorenson, R. C. 1973. *Adolescent Sexuality in Contemporary America.* New York: World Publishing.

Stanley v. State of Illinois. 92 S.Ct. 1208, 1972.

Tyrer, L. B. and Josimovich, J. 1977. Contraception in teenagers. *Clin. Obstet. Gynecol.* 20:651–663.

Urban and Rural Systems Associates. 1976. *Improving Family Planning Services for Teenagers.* Final report submitted to Office of the Assistant Secretary for Planning and Evaluation/Health. DHEW Contract #HEW-OS 74 304, June.

Vener, A. and Stewart, C. 1974. Adolescent sexual behavior in middle America revisited: 1970–1973. *J. Marr. Fam.* 36(4):728–735.

Westoff, C. F. 1976. Trends in contraceptive practice: 1965–1973. *Fam. Plann. Perspect.* 8(2):54–57.

Zabin, L. S., Kantner, J. F. and Zelnik, M. 1979. The risk of adolescent pregnancy in the first months of intercourse. *Fam. Plann. Perspect.* 11(4):215–222.

Zackler, J. and Brandstandt, W. 1975. *The Teenage Pregnancy Girl.* Springfield, Illinois: Charles C Thomas.

Zelnik, M. and Kantner, J. F. 1978. Contraceptive patterns and premarital pregnancy among women aged 15–19 in 1976. *Fam. Plann. Perspect.* 10:135–142.

11

A Mental Health Program
for Adolescent Parents

CARLOS SALGUERO, NANCY SCHLESINGER, AND EDILMA YEARWOOD

The complex problem of teenage pregnancy continues to be of significant concern to medical and mental health professionals, educators, and policymakers at national and state levels for very good reasons. Pregnancy triggers a series of events which bear serious consequences for the youngster and her offspring from a medical, psychological, and sociological point of view.

In response to the need for controlling and reducing the incidence of pregnancies in this young age group, health, educational, and social agencies have developed a variety of programs to educate and meet the needs of sexually active adolescents. Many concentrate on birth control counseling for those sexually active adolescents at high risk for pregnancy, and abortion counseling for the pregnant ones. Hospitals and health agencies provide services for childbearing teenagers as part of their regular prenatal services. Services for girls in lower socioeconomic groups tend to focus on the later stages of the prenatal and postnatal period. After the baby is born, active follow-up very often does not take place, and agencies learn about the young mother when she again requests prenatal services.

From an educational point of view, there has been an expansion of programs that enable the adolescent mother to return to school, improve her employment opportunities, or get assistance with her medical, psychological, and social needs. According to Baldwin (1976) and the Alan Guttmacher Institute (1976), pregnancy continues to be the most frequent cause of adolescent school drop-out.

181

For the adolescent, the psychological trauma of pregnancy with its disruptive effect on psychosexual development, object relationships, and identity formation, needs careful attention because it will determine the quality of life choices and the manner in which the girl will achieve her ego ideal. It will also have a direct effect on her relationship to her infant, her degree of attachment to him/her, and her ability to view him/her as separate from herself. Thus, it will also have an effect on her child's intellectual and affective development (see Chapters 7 and 8, this volume).

Pregnant adolescents need optimal medical care and educational and social supports on a long-term basis if they are to achieve their fullest potential. Hospital, school, and social agency-based Adolescent Pregnancy Programs have been implemented to help this population; yet very few programs have a specific mental health component to continuously assess and assist pregnant adolescents and adolescent mothers and their children in their developmental needs and to help the young mother develop a better understanding of her child and herself as both continue to grow and relate to each other. To highlight this need, Salguero et al (1980) reported on how adolescents differ among themselves in their attitudes toward their pregnancies and their babies.

The following is a description of a comprehensive adolescent pregnancy program developed by the Mental Health Services Department of the Hill Health Center. This was arranged to meet the psychological, social, and health needs of sexually active and pregnant adolescents and adolescent mothers and their children who live in a low income neighborhood of New Haven, Connecticut.

THE COMMUNITY

Roughly triangular in shape, the densely populated catchment area known as the Hill community covers about two square miles; poverty is evident in the neighborhood. Burned buildings and vacant lots are a common sight. Recreational facilities and green areas are practically nonexistent. Children and adolescents grow up in an ambience in which they feel ostracized and trapped by a system that provides few healthy outlets; at the same time, the youngsters are exposed to all the negative elements of slum living, such as high unemployment, abundant street drugs, and apartment overcrowding. The population of this community is 21,000 according to the 1970 United States census. Recent city estimates place it at 24,000, made up of 40 percent blacks, 30 percent Hispanics, and 30 percent whites. Thirty-nine percent of this population is comprised of children and adolescents aged 12 to 18. Over one third of the families receive state or city welfare. The unemployment rate is very high for adolescents.

THE HILL HEALTH CENTER

The Hill Health Center is a community-controlled health facility that provides comprehensive health services to the Hill community. This is accomplished by three clinical teams made up of physicians (pediatricians, internists, and obstetricians), nurses (public health, pediatric, and family practitioners), community health workers, nutritionists, dentists, and mental health specialists (child psychiatrists, social workers, special education teachers, and psychologists). The number of persons presently enrolled at the Center is 13,000. A pharmacy and a laboratory provide support services. Hospital services are provided by Yale-New Haven Hospital, six blocks away from the Center. The local middle and high schools are also within walking distance.

The Teenage Pregnancy and Parenting Program (TAPPP) was developed by the Center's Mental Health Services Department to coordinate the services offered by the Hill Health Center to sexually active, pregnant adolescents and young mothers and their children in a continuous and timely manner through an extended period of time ranging from the time the adolescent requests a pregnancy test to the time her child becomes four years old. At the same time, the mental health staff provide the adolescent with continuous emotional support and practical assistance with the ongoing adjustments they must make regarding themselves, their changing relationships to others, and the demands made by the community.

The decision by the staff to develop such services was due to their observation that these adolescents felt emotionally overwhelmed by their pregnancy and later on by the demands made by their infants, often their second child. Central to our decision to intervene therapeutically was the question whether many of our adolescent mothers were psychologically prepared for motherhood, a necessary condition for optimal maternal-infant attachment to take place. Unfortunately, not all the adolescents who participated in the program were ready for motherhood. As Provence, Naylor, and Solnit (1977) said, taking good care of, and loving, a baby requires more psychological ingredients than a biological relationship between a mother and her baby. Thus, the staff felt that by protecting the often fragile mother-infant bond, infants would be at lesser risk for situations that lead to child abuse, neglect, and failure-to-thrive.

The conditions for sexually active adolescents were equally precarious. The number of adolescents from the local high school who requested pregnancy tests at the Hill Health Center was very high. For example, in 1976, of 46 adolescents who had become pregnant, 18 had had previous negative pregnancy tests. Misconceptions and ignorance of birth control and human sexuality were, and continue to be, widespread. More importantly, while many adolescents remained in school after they became pregnant, many others dropped out.

From a health point of view, pregnant adolescents tended to use the Center's prenatal services (obstetrics/gynecology, nutrition, dental, prenatal classes, etc.) during the third trimester and immediately after delivery with very little follow-up.

From a psychological point of view, many of the adolescents appeared depressed and confused, and often were ambivalent about acceptance of their future offspring. Young mothers felt overwhelmed by the new babies' needs and their new mothering responsibilities. Intensive primary and secondary prevention efforts were clearly needed. Although individual psychological factors played a role in the decision for a girl to get pregnant, the increase in the number of pregnancies, especially for the group aged 15 years and under in 1976, indicated that other factors played a key role, such as increase in sexual activity and changing sexual standards, few opportunities for personal fulfillment, and other social and cultural factors. In a community in which few sublimatory channels exist, sexual activity is resorted to by teenagers to fulfill by instant gratification their current needs, and to raise their low self-esteem by having a baby that they believe can love them, rather than planning for a future clouded with uncertainties and problems.

A comprehensive program like TAPPP, designed for an inner-city, low income, high risk population, is feasible because of the Hill Health Center's unique delivery of health care services in which several disciplines, working in teams, provide the necessary services and supports around which the coordination of services was developed. The adolescent and her family are usually known to the health team members. Part of the Center's strategy of health care delivery is their outreach programs, through which any clinical member of the team may make a home or a school visit. The active home visits are welcomed by families and prevent, to a large measure, the client's tendency to miss appointments; they also strengthen the relationship between the family and the Center. On the other hand, this family-Center relationship was viewed with suspicion by our teenage population since they questioned the Center's ability to maintain confidentiality about their visits, especially when they requested birth control, pregnancy tests, or abortion counselling. For this reason, TAPPP counseling services were also designed to be delivered in settings which are separated geographically from the Center.

TAPPP was initiated in 1976 by the Mental Health Services department senior social worker along with the help of work-study students from Yale University. Due to financial constraints, the program functioned on a limited basis until October 1977, when additional funds for a demonstration grant were secured through the Administration of Children, Youth and Families (ACYF) of the Department of Health, Education, and Welfare. This funding enabled the program to expand and include a coordinator, social worker, public health nurse, two community health workers, and a secretary. This new staff, together with the existing Mental Health Services Department staff, the teams, and the full array of medical and health professionals at the Hill Health Center, coordinated the comprehensive services in a more meaningful fashion.

COMPREHENSIVE SERVICES

The word "comprehensive" needs further definition. We define comprehensive programs as those that directly coordinate medical, social, and educational services for sexually active, pregnant, and childbearing adolescents until the mother and child are no longer at risk for pregnancy-related factors, and can be followed adequately by local, state, and federal agencies. The Program Directory of the National Alliance with School-Age Parents (1976) lists only 54 (4.8 percent) services of 1,132 classified programs in the directory as having the three components: health, education, and social services.

TAPPP's conceptual framework of service delivery translates research and clinical findings into a truly comprehensive community program. It intervenes at the level of the sexually active, childbearing, and child-rearing adolescent. Within each of these stages, goals are established that are of particular significance for that segment of the population. Working in concert with other agencies, using a variety of educational and counseling strategies, TAPPP aims at preventing pregnancy in a population defined as being at high risk for this event. It protects the physical and emotional well-being of the expectant mother and her future offspring while efforts are made to prevent school dropout. The young mother and her infant are provided with optimal protection by a series of intensive health, educational, and mental health services in which the fostering of a positive mother-infant bond and the prevention of child abuse and neglect are major subgoals.

The program addresses itself to the individual adolescent's developmental needs and provides the types of support (where and when) needed since the services are continuous and individualized throughout. There are no criteria for selection. The adolescent enters the program when she wants to find out if she is pregnant. By reaching out to the adolescent at different stages of her contacts with the Center, the program enhances the adolescent's use of the Hill Health Center services and provides the staff to assist her in her needs.

DESCRIPTION OF THE PROGRAM

The adolescent enters the program when she requests a pregnancy test, either through self-referral or by another person, usually a staff member from the Center. An average of 16 adolescents request pregnancy tests each month.

The results of the test are shared in a private, confidential counseling session with the Mental Health Services rotating social worker for that day.

If the pregnancy test has a negative result, the social worker, after determining the possible causes that led to the request for the pregnancy test, counsels the adolescent about preventing a future pregnancy. This includes birth control counseling, and, when required, social and therapeutic intervention. Coordination with other Hill Health Center services, such as obstetrics/gynecology, is made available to the adolescent with appropriate follow-up.

If the pregnancy test has a positive finding; intensive counseling is provided in order to help the adolescent reach a decision whether to continue with her pregnancy or choose an abortion. If she opts for abortion, the social worker may accompany and assist the adolescent through the abortion procedures. Close follow-up is provided until it is felt that the adolescent is doing well from an emotional and physical point of view.

If the adolescent decides to continue with her pregnancy, the social worker becomes her primary worker and will continue to follow the adolescent through her pregnancy and motherhood to insure continuity of care until the child and mother graduate from the program. This takes place when the child is four years old and has access to regular or specialized federal- or state-funded programs.

Any pregnant girl who did not have a pregnancy test at the Center, or who has just moved to the area, may join the program when she seeks prenatal care for the first time. In some cases, another staff member from the Center, usually a public health nurse or community health worker from the team, becomes the adolescent's primary worker, especially when a relationship already exists between the staff member and the adolescent.

The concept of the primary worker is the basis for the unique nature of TAPPP follow-up and is central to the delivery of mental health-oriented services for adolescent mothers. The primary worker insures coordination of services, with follow-up and outreach if a breakdown occurs. The primary worker is the advocate for the adolescent within the Health Center's system and in the community. Through this relationship, she may learn of the adolescent's home situation, educational plans, relationships with significant others, and feelings about her pregnancy and ensuing motherhood. Knowledge about infant care and parenting skills may also be assessed. The development of a primary worker-client relationship enables the worker to make predictions regarding the future for the young mother and her infant.

The TAPP Program is especially concerned with the "at risk" designation identified by the primary worker at regular intervals beginning with the seventh month of pregnancy and continuing through the infant's first four years (see Appendix for definition of at risk designation.) Bimonthly case conferences, attended by the adolescent's primary worker, TAPPP, and other Hill Health

Center staff working with the adolescent, are structured so that all prenatal cases are reviewed at the seventh month, immediately after delivery, at three-month intervals during the infant's first year, and continuing at six-month intervals until the fourth year. The decision to review all cases going to term at the seventh month of pregnancy is based on Bibring's (1959) clinical observations on the "quickening" phenomenon which occurs around the 20th week of pregnancy. The baby's first movements bring to the expectant mother an awareness that there is a new distinct object within herself which will continue to grow in her body until delivery while she herself continues to experience extensive body changes. The emotional adjustment to this new perception of herself and her baby will affect the mother's attachment and relationship to her baby. The seventh month thus provides the staff with an opportunity to review the adolescent's attitude toward her baby, her psychological and health status, her relationship toward her boyfriend and family, and her economic and social situation. After review of these and other related factors, the staff decide the type and intensity of intervention most appropriate in each case during the remainder of the pregnancy, delivery, and after the adolescent and her baby return home.

With the case review at the seventh month, the client is considered part of the Infant Stimulation Program (ISP), the component of TAPPP focused on working with adolescent parents and their infants. Once she is part of ISP, the adolescent will be introduced to her team's public health nurse and will have the opportunity to become involved with the Parent-Infant Center.

The ISP offers the full range of Hill Health Center services to the adolescent and her infant. Each infant, has a regular physical examination at two weeks, six weeks, three months, six months, and 12 months in the first year and two regular physical examinations each year until age four. These visits are usually well coordinated with visits to the nutritionist, Women, Infant, and Children Program, and TAPPP primary worker. The physical layout of the Hill Health Center also enables TAPPP to follow-up on unscheduled medical visits, not unusual when an infant is involved. Screening and laboratory tests for disease, immunizations, and height and weight measurement tables are carefully recorded. Developmental screening is performed at the ninth month and second year using the Yale Child Study Center Developmental Assessment Scale.

Continuous assessment is made of the relationship between the young mother and her child and active intervention is made by TAPPP and Hill Health Center staff to ameliorate or eliminate those factors that create stress in the mother-infant dyad, while helping to foster a healthy relationship. While the emphasis of the intervention is directed towards mother-infant interaction, a great deal of attention is also focused on assisting the young mother to continue her own development. This includes addressing issues such as postponement of the second pregnancy, continuation of her education, and helping to make arrangements for child care to reduce social isolation and allow the adolescent to participate in peer group activities. The mental health of the adolescent mother is thus considered crucial for the positive growth of both mother and infant.

THE PARENT-INFANT CENTER

A continuation of the ISP is the Parent-Infant Center (PIC). Originally, it was conceived as a therapeutic program to work with adolescent mothers whose infants are believed to be at high risk for neglect and/or abuse. It has widened its focus to teach parenting skills to any pregnant adolescent who wishes to participate in it.

At their seventh month of pregnancy, all interested adolescents are introduced by their primary worker to the PIC staff. In order to prepare her for the upcoming delivery and the establishment of her relationship with her infant, the adolescent participates in class exercises, tours the hospital delivery room, and attends workshops on breast-feeding, safety, toys, parenting, child development, health care, etc. The emphasis is on helping the adolescent develop a positive attitude toward her baby. Her PIC involvement terminates when the baby is three months old and the adolescent continues in the TAPP Program under the watchful eye of the primary worker and other Hill Health Center staff.

If it appears that the adolescent has conflicts about her future relationship to her baby at the seventh month review, or there are clear indications that her attitude toward the fetus is negative and rejecting, the adolescent is formally referred to the therapeutic component of the PIC program. The goal in this case is to provide therapeutic intervention to deal with the factors responsible for the adolescent's difficulties. The program follows the adolescent mother during the infant's first year of life. While the primary worker continues to play an important therapeutic role, the adolescent is assigned to a PIC staff member who will work with the young mother and her infant at the Center in individual and group activities. If this is not possible, the staff continues the therapeutic work in a homebound plan. Both the primary worker and PIC staff monitor the progress the adolescent is making in the program at the regular bimonthly meetings.

PREVENTIVE EFFORTS IN THE COMMUNITY

The goal of reducing the incidence of adolescent pregnancy is difficult to reach since the factors that lead to pregnancy are varied and complex, especially in our catchment area where ethnic, social, and psychological factors play a major role in maintaining a high incidence and prevalence of adolescent pregnancies. Some studies, such as that by Goldfarb et al (1977), have begun to identify those adolescents that are susceptible to pregnancy. In their study, the authors found that (1) the susceptible adolescent is not at grade level and shows signs generally of having a poor and disrupted academic record, (2) an adolescent from a larger family is more susceptible than an adolescent from a smaller family, and (3) sex education introduced at a late age and by a nonfamily member increases the likelihood of susceptibility.

Data analysis of 114 teenagers from our community, seen in our program, gives a profile of the typical TAPPP client: she is most likely to be black (60.9 percent) and single (74.5 percent), may or may not be in school (52.7 percent in school), lives with her family (62 percent), and is not using birth control (70 percent). A strong objective implemented by TAPPP is to provide the adolescent with as much information as possible about health, human sexuality, and contraceptive counseling through pamphlets developed by the program, a newspaper written by adolescents under the auspices of the Hill Health Center, health fairs, and individual counseling. TAPPP is also coordinating its work with other agencies and institutions with similar concerns who are trying to accomplish related goals with sexually active adolescents, pregnant adolescents, and young mothers. Together with the Yale Child Study Center and the local high school, the Hill Health Center has established the Teenage Health Education and Parenting Consortium to prevent adolescents from dropping out because of pregnancy and to facilitate their return after delivery by providing them with a specialized parenting curriculum. It also has provided workshops for the school faculty to sensitize them to the problems the adolescents face in the community. The need to coordinate services for sexually active adolescents in New Haven has led the Hill Health Center to provide free pregnancy testing for any adolescent in New Haven who is eligible for Title XX. Adolescents thus receive contraceptive and pregnancy counseling; if more help is needed, other community agencies have formally agreed to continue working with them.

COMMENTS

The success of an adolescent pregnancy program lies in its ability to conceptualize a philosophy of approach translatable into viable program objectives reached in a comprehensive approach or in the program's being a component of a system of linkages to help the adolescent. In the case of the Teenage Pregnancy Program, the approach is a developmental one, and one which addresses itself to a key concept—the protection of the emotional well-being of both the mother and her child. On that basis, the program assists female adolescents by taking into account their stage of psychological development, ego strengths, and object relationships, and, most importantly, the quality of their relationship to their infant and families. Once a psychosocial profile has been established, the program assists the adolescent in a timely manner and provides her with the practical and emotional support needed to cope with the many implications of pregnancy.

A thorough knowledge of the girl's psychic development at the time of conception is needed as well as an understanding of those community pressures which put her at high risk for pregnancy, such as overcrowding, the birth of a baby in the family, problems with her mother, peers or sisters getting pregnant, etc. It must be kept in mind, however, that although the factors that lead an adolescent girl to become pregnant are complex, how she will experience it psychologically and adjust to it depend very much on whether she is in her early, mid, or late stage of adolescence (see Chapters 4 and 8, this volume). The primary worker, who follows the adolescent through an extended period of time, is in the ideal position to assess the adolescent's strengths, concerns, and difficulties and to provide her with the type of practical and emotional support to foster her and her child's development. Thus, a 17-year-old adolescent who had been abused as a child, and who expressed fears of not being able to attach to her infant just delivered through a Caesarean section, was able to do so when her primary worker helped her to deal with her feelings of abuse and worked with the hospital staff to facilitate attachment behaviors. In the same manner, assistance and support is crucial during the child's stage of separation-individuation, when the toddler's own quest for autonomy and independence raises many angry and competitive feelings from the 14- to 15-year-old adolescent mother who is struggling with her own conflicts of separation from her mother and the absence of her own father and boyfriend.

An adolescent pregnancy program must address itself to the developmental needs of the pregnant adolescent and, later, the young mother and her child. The model presented in this chapter uses a developmental approach as its philosophy of intervention.

A program, no matter how limited or comprehensive, will only be successful if it can measure consistently the goals it has set out to accomplish. Some objectives are more tangible than others. Jekel (1975) and Klerman (1979) strongly recommended that a program must identify the population to be studied and determine if the established objectives will benefit most of the population. The program's objectives should be made specific in measurable terms in at least three areas: the target population, the services offered, and the outcomes expected. The longer the follow-up of the new parents and their children, the better. For example, TAPPP reached some desired health goals by increasing the number of adolescents receiving prenatal care in the first trimester of pregnancy (Table 1) by lowering the prematurity rate to less than one percent (compared with the previous rate of 16 percent in 1976), and by attaining a very low number of pregnancy and delivery complications. Most comprehensive programs

Table 1.   Trimester of Prenatal Care Initiation

| Trimester | TAPPP Clients (Number) | |
| | 1976 (n = 52) | 1978 (n = 40) |
	N (%)	N (%)
1st Trimester	10(19)	24(60)
2nd Trimester	16(31)	7(18)
3rd Trimester	26(50)	9(22)

have been able to replicate these goals. In addition, the number of adolescent mothers reported for child abuse has dropped to only one in 1977 and 1978 as compared with six in the year 1976.

Our goal to help adolescents return to school has been more difficult to reach. More than 50 percent of the black mothers participating in our program have been able to return to school or work while few Hispanics were able to do so. Hispanic mothers, in general, do not view themselves as "students" but as mothers to their infants who, therefore, must stay home. Other common factors that prevent young mothers from returning to school are the absence of subsidized day care programs or the "red tape" that adolescents must deal with to obtain subsidies. Schools also do not offer flexible schedules to facilitate the adolescent's return to school.

The most important goal for programs with a school component is to prevent school drop-out, which is more common in girls who become pregnant as they enter the ninth grade, as well as to help the young mother return to school, graduate, and successfully enter the job market. Another important and related goal is the prevention of repeat pregnancy. Repeat pregnancies indicate that a young mother will not only find it more difficult to cope with educational and working demands, but that she has a greater chance of remaining in or entering the welfare system and of remaining poor. In a study of teenage pregnancy and welfare dependency, Moore (1978) reported that in 1975 about half of the funds distributed to AFDC households ($4.65 billion of $9.4 billion disbursed) went to women who had had their first child during their teen years. The study showed early childbearers to be "consistently more likely to need AFDC support than women of the age who postponed childbearing."

Our definition and description of a "comprehensive" program is important because it has a specific meaning for the Department of Health, Education, and Welfare. In 1977, Senator Kennedy introduced a new bill: The Adolescent Health Services and Pregnancy Prevention and Care Act of 1978. Congressmen John Brademas and Paul Rogers introduced a companion bill. The legislation reached final passage on October 14, 1978, when it was included as

Titles VI, VII, and VIII of the Health Services and Centers amendments of 1978. It became Public Law 95-626 on November 10, 1978. In 1979, the Office of Adolescent Pregnancy Programs (OAPP) was established. Comprehensive programs funded by this office must offer pregnancy testing, family planning services, primary and preventive health services, nutrition information and counseling, referral for screening and treatment of venereal disease, appropriate pediatric care, educational services in sexuality and family life, educational and vocational services, adoption counseling and referral services, and other health services. Other supplemental services that may be required are child care, consumer education and homemaking counseling for extended family members, transportation, and other essential services.

Many questions remain unanswered. Some of them will only become more evident over an extended period of observation. For example, in spite of program efforts, we know so little about the fathers and the effect the relative lack of male role models within the family will have on the young infant's development (see Chapter 5, this volume).

In spite of the successes reported by some teenage programs in different areas of prevention, much remains to be learned about adolescents. Our concept of "help" is viewed suspiciously by many of them. Agencies often tend to be judgmental if not punitive when they seek help. In studying the help-seeking behaviors among adolescent parents, Cannon-Bonventre and Kahn (1979) reported that the parents in their study often felt forced into an adversary relationship with service agencies in that they were made to feel as though they were getting help in the form of some special favor or as a handout. A number of teenage parents found themselves in the uncomfortable position of simultaneously being treated as children and being expected to undertake adult roles. Programs should therefore act as advocates for the adolescents and their children whom they serve by making efforts to change and redirect community attitudes to ensure the psychosocial, physical, and emotional well-being of this special population.

SUMMARY

The Teenage Pregnancy and Parenting Program developed by the Mental Health Department of a neighborhood health center is an example of a comprehensive delivery of services to sexually active, pregnant and childbearing adolescents. It is the opinion of the authors that by understanding the adolescent's developmental needs during critical periods of her pregnancy and motherhood, a primary worker and the team can effectively assist her in a timely manner while ensuring the infant's emotional well-being. This chapter describes the program and how some of its goals were reached with the hope that other programs can benefit from our experience.

APPENDIX

Minimal Risk Child: A child considered under this category suffers only from minor or no medical problems at all. His physical and emotional development are within normal limits for his age. His mother is in tune with his needs and keeps all Hill Health Center appointments for herself and her child. She also makes appropriate plans for both and is coping well with the stresses of young motherhood. She receives or avails herself of emotional and social supports when needed.

Moderate Risk Child: This is a child who suffers from a reversible medical condition and/or developmental interference or delay. Another criterion for moderate risk is a child whose mother cannot cope successfully with the demanding tasks of motherhood due to ongoing personal, family, or social problems. These problems interfere with the mother's ability to care optimally for her child, manifested by not keeping all her Hill Health Center appointments for herself and her child and by often feeling overwhelmed by her child's demands. The young mother expresses positive feelings towards her child.

High Risk Child: A child who is suffering from a serious medical condition is at high risk for failure to thrive, child abuse, and neglect when his mother is definitely not coping with her mothering responsibilities. This may be due to serious problems of a personal, family, or social nature which have led to a negative perception of herself and her infant, expression of negative feelings, total failure to keep appointments, and poor child care. A child can also be at high risk when his mother is facing acute problems that totally interfere with her ability to relate to her baby. By giving an at-risk designation to each case, it is felt that therapeutic strategies to help the young mothers can be better directed, especially in cases considered at high risk.

ACKNOWLEDGMENT

This work was supported by Grant 90-C-1337 from the Administration for Children, Youth and Families.

REFERENCES

Alan Guttmacher Institute. 1976. *Eleven Million Teenagers: What Can Be Done About the Epidemic of Adolescent Pregnancies in the United States?* New York: Planned Parenthood Federation of America.

Baldwin, W. 1976. Adolescent pregnancy and childbearing—growing concerns for Americans. *Popul. Bull.* 31 (2).

Bibring, G. 1959. Some considerations of the psychological processes of pregnancy. *Psychoanal. Study Child* 14:113–121.

Cannon-Bonventre, K. and Kahn, J. 1979. *The Ecology of Help-Seeking Behavior Among Adolescent Parents.* Report prepared for Administration for Children, Youth and Families.

Goldfarb, J., Mumford, D., Schum, D., Smith, P., Flowers, C. and Schum, C. 1977. An attempt to detect "pregnancy susceptibility" in indigent adolescent girls. *J. Youth Adol.* 6(1):127–143.

Jekel, J. 1975. Appraising programs for school-age parents. Design problems. *Eval. Health Profess.* 1:55–70.

Klerman, L. 1979. Evaluating service programs for school-age parents. *J. School Health* 45:296–300.

Moore, K. 1978. Teenage childbirth and welfare dependency. *Fam. Plann. Perspect.* 10(4):233–235.

National Alliance Concerned with School-Age Parents. 1976. *National Directory of Services for School-Age Parents.* Washington, DC.

Provence, S., Naylor, P., and Solnit, A. 1977. *The Challenge of Day Care.* New Haven, Connecticut: Yale University Press.

Salguero, C., Yearwood, E., Phillips, E. and Schlesinger, N. 1980. Studies of infants at risk and their adolescent mothers. *Adol. Psychiatry* 8:404–421.

Implications for Programs

12

Funding for Pregnant Adolescents: A Legislative History

KATHLEEN RUDD SCHARF

INTRODUCTION

Twenty years ago, caring for unmarried pregnant adolescents was largely the province of voluntary social agencies. America viewed nonmarital childbearing as deviant behavior, and a particularly contagious form of deviance at that. The teenage birthrate was, in fact, higher than it is today: 90 of every 1,000 young women under twenty gave birth in the late 1950s, while only 58 out of every 1,000 did so in the middle 1970s (Alan Guttmacher Institute, 1976). Some socioeconomic strata and cultural groups were more tolerant of visible single parenthood than others, but most were grateful to agencies like the Salvation Army and the Florence Crittenden League for dealing quietly with "wayward girls." Middle class girls who became pregnant (and did not marry) received adequate physical care, returning to their families without outward physical stigmata. The national linkage of agencies permitted respectable girls to leave for a "stay with relatives" in another city whose maternity home kept them safe from chance discovery.

By the late 1950s, a high percentage of infants born to maternity home residents were given up for adoption, through the homes themselves or through allied agencies (for example, Crittenden Hastings House, 1978). Previous motherhood could be hidden from husbands and other associates in later years, and infertile couples enjoyed a relatively good chance of adopting a healthy white infant. Everyone involved could rest assured that unmarried mothers would learn, though direct instruction and indirect evidence, that nonmarital sex and its sequelae were unacceptable.

Many forces have combined to transform the landscape of adolescent pregnancy services. The historical trend away from voluntarism toward public sector management of social services certainly has affected patterns of contribution and resort, but the changes in attitude and behavior we have come to call the "sexual revolution" of the 1960s have been much more important.

Begging the question of origin, the results are manifest. The development of the oral contraceptive and the intraurerine device has allowed many sexually active persons to assume that sex and reproduction can be separated at will. The widening legal availability of abortions has extended the expectation of absolute reproductive control, and adolescents whose chief concerns are secrecy and/or continuity of life planning resort more frequently to abortion than they could or would have 20 years ago. More adolescent pregnancies are being terminated by abortion, and fewer adolescent births lead to adoption. The revolution among sexually active adolescents seems to consist of several phenomena: more sexual activity, more contraception, more pregnancies, more abortions, fewer births, fewer "shotgun" marriages, and fewer adoptions. A widely used statistical abstract of adolescent sexual and reproductive behavior reports the following numerical breakdown for 1974: one million American teenagers became pregnant, and 600,000 of these pregnancies resulted in live births. (At the same time, perhaps 12 million US teenagers were sexually active.) However, more than half (approximately 382,000) of these births were to married mothers, and about three quarters of the marital births were *postmaritally* conceived (Alan Guttmacher Institute, 1976).

In fact, the widespread expression of concern about "teenage pregnancy" tends to focus on the very real problem of a minority of pregnant adolescents—those who give birth out of wedlock. Only about 20 percent of conceptions among girls under 20 years of age in 1974 yielded out-of-wedlock births, but 87.4 percent, or about 193,000, of these babies remained with their biological mother (Alan Guttmacher Institute, 1976). It is important to keep this breakdown of statistics in mind when considering statements about an "epidemic of adolescent pregnancies."

As technical aids and societal attitudes combined to facilitate changes in adolescent sexual and reproductive behavior, pregnant adolescents gained some legal rights as well. Despite attempts to legally mandate parental consent or consultation, minors can obtain abortions at their own request in most parts of the country. A 1971 Federal court ruling, Ordway v. Hargraves, forced public schools to allow pregnant students to attend regular classes. This reduced forced discontinuities in education, while in a sense encouraging school districts which prefer to sequester pregnant students to provide special programs more attractive than the normal school curriculum.

These shifts in norms, laws, and numbers have affected the providers of social and medical services tremendously. Some older voluntary agencies have adapted to the changing needs and expectations of their clients by establishing pregnancy counseling, abortion, and nonresidential maternity services. Embroidery lessons have given way to child development, nutrition, and parenting classes. There is greater attention to postnatal planning for mother and child. Biological fathers have started to receive some attention. Nationally, however, private agencies no longer dominate the field. Some areas now have service centers for childbearing adolescents that combine the services of federal, state, city, school, and private entities, but many regions of the country lack coordinated services and young mothers must seek prenatal and postnatal care piecemeal. It is to this welter of changed demands and expectations that individuals and agencies reacted in the early 1970s by forming a loose "adolescent pregnancy lobby."

THE ADOLESCENT PREGNANCY LOBBY

For several years the "adolescent pregnancy lobby" called for (1) better funding and (2) better coordination and rationalization of services for childbearing adolescents. These voices included organizations such as the National Alliance Concerned for School-Age Parents (NACSAP), Planned Parenthood, Zero Population Growth (ZPG), and Eunice Kennedy Shriver of the Joseph P. Kennedy, Jr. Foundation. Shriver's brother, Senator Edward Kennedy of Massachusetts, began hearings on teenage pregnancy and childbearing in 1974, featuring representatives of NACSAP, the Kennedy Foundation, and other entities. Witnesses testified to the numerical medical and social seriousness of adolescent childbearing, and the inadequacies of the poorly funded and badly coordinated social services charged with ministering to young parents. The political clout of these observers was especially limited in a year of recession by the fact that they were asking for expensive services to nonvoting recipients.

THE CARTER ADOLESCENT PREGNANCY INITIATIVE

Two years later, advocates of expanded services to adolescent parents received a political boost from an unexpected quarter. Both presidential candidates were summoned before the US Conference of Bishops, and Democratic candidate Jimmy Carter joined his Republican opponent Gerald Ford in agreeing with the Roman Catholic bishops' stand against induced abortion. Carter understood the temper of his liberal political support well enough to stop short of advocating an antiabortion "right to life" amendment to the Constitution, but reacted to pressure from the bishops and other antiabortion questioners by stating a personal preference for "alternatives" to abortion, particularly for adolescents. After Carter's election, his appointee as Secretary of the Department of Health, Education, and Welfare (DHEW), Joseph A. Califano, Jr., echoed the President's preference for "alternatives" to abortion during his Senate confirmation hearings.

By May 1977, Califano had instructed his deputies at DHEW to look into the state of American approaches to adolescent childbearing; the Carter administration had already raised the family planning budget requests of the previous administration. Reports submitted to Califano described chaos in most areas of the country, with services for sexually active and childbearing adolescents as ill defined and badly coordinated as witnesses at Senator Kennedy's 1974 hearings had claimed. Califano's assistants had also visited comprehensive projects, such as The Door in New York City, and the Secretary himself was influenced by his personal friends, the Shrivers, to admire a comprehensive program at Johns Hopkins in Baltimore funded by the Kennedy Foundation.

CONGRESSIONAL ACTION

In February 1978, the House Select Committee on Population held hearings on adolescent childbearing and the extent of existing services for young parents. Those who testified agreed with each other that an "epidemic" of teenage childbearing existed, that a great outpouring of money was needed to alleviate the social, physical, and economic problems of young parents, and that a federal effort was required to intervene in such a massive, expensive set of problems. Witnesses disagreed, however, over the specific priorities of ideal programs. As had long been the case, the basically liberal, prochoice organizations were inclined to emphasize pregnancy counseling and to assume that abortion was often the preferable response to an adolescent pregnancy, while more conservative, prolife organizations like the Kennedy Foundation supported "moral development" guidance for nonpregnant adolescents and physical supports for childbearers.

Finally, on April 13, the Carter administration bill arrived in Congress. The "Adolescent Health, Services and Pregnancy Prevention and Care Act of 1978" involved an administration request for a $60 million funding level. At the same time, Secretary Califano announced that he had appointed Lulu Mae Nix, director of the only statewide program for adolescent childbearers (in Delaware), to coordinate all future DHEW efforts to provide such services. The bill was vague, calling for "linkages" between services, "expansion" of services, and the promotion of "innovative" approaches to the problems of adolescent parents. A fairly typical report in a prochoice newsletter was glum:

> Introduced in the Senate as S.2910 and in the House as H.R.12146, the legislation already is off to a bad start politically. The rules of Congress

require committees to report out new legislation such as this by May 15 if there is to be a vote on it in either the Senate or the House. The Senate hearings will come after that deadline, and the House has not set hearing dates. That means the committees will have to seek waivers of the reporting deadlines.

While the bill is the kind of "motherhood and apple pie" legislation that is hard for Congress to reject—especially in an election year—political support for it is not solid, either. In the House, it was introduced only "at the request" of the Administration by Rep. Paul Rogers, chairman of the Commerce subcommittee on health and the environment, and Rep. John Brademas, chairman of the Education and Labor subcommittee on select education (Zero Population Growth, 1978).

ADOLESCENT PREGNANCY LOBBY REACTIONS

Hearings were held by the Senate Committee on Human Resources in June and July, 1978. Many advocates of expanded federal involvement in adolescent services found the Administration bill unacceptable, but their criticisms were muted by a desire to encourage the executive and legislative branches to continue to move quickly and generously. Those who testified during the 1978 hearings were cautiously critical, concerned with the vagueness of the draft bill and the extent to which it would give DHEW broad power to determine funding priorities through the regulation-writing process (Senate Committee on Human Resources, 1978a, 1978b). Washington population hands were reminded of Secretary Califano's service in the Johnson administration, when large budgets and nebulous legislative language maximized federal control over social programs. In this context, Secretary Califano's antiabortion statements and the temper of Congress led prochoice lobbyists to fear the fate of their own priorities at the hands of DHEW regulation and guideline writers; indeed, at this point Congress had begun passing an annual antiabortion "Hyde Amendment" to the Federal Medicaid appropriation, and DHEW under Califano was interpreting Congressional intent rather strictly through its Medicaid abortion regulations. Although the bill seemed to many interested parties to favor maternity care to the detriment of pregnancy prevention, there was also support for the belief that a pregnancy care emphasis could serve to supplement existing federal family planning programs while an over-broad bill might serve as an excuse for Congressional cutbacks in those programs. Those who favored this latter strategy, such as Peters Willson of Zero Population Growth, felt that it was more useful to avoid arguing over prevention components versus service components, and to concentrate instead on dividing federal funds between services for the "never-pregnant" and "already-pregnant" client.

THE PROFILE/PROCHOICE COALITION

As hearings and bill markups proceeded, the Kennedy Foundation arranged for a meeting between prolife and prochoice lobbyists interested in funding for childbearing adolescents. The first attempts at forming an adolescent childbearing coalition went slowly; the erstwhile legislative opponents were generally "too nervous to do much," as one member observed. Prochoice members included Willson of ZPG and representatives of the National Alliance Concerned for School-Age Parents; prolife members included Marjory Mecklenburg of American Citizens Concerned for Life, Inc., Thea Barron of the National Right to Life Committee, and Eunice Kennedy Shriver of the Kennedy Foundation. Meanwhile, hearings on the Carter bill were still dealing with vague goals, and members of the nascent coalition were concerned that what they saw as real issues in the provision of care for adolescent childbearers would not come up. In late summer of 1978, the coalition tried again, members now trying to avoid the fatally divisive issues of abortion counseling and abortion provision. A conciliatory role was taken by Maris Vinovskis, a population historian and demographer acting as assistant staff director of the now-defunct House Select Committee on Population. Vinovskis in particular wished to facilitate the definition of an effective funding approach acceptable to both prochoice and prolife activitists. He was uniquely suited to his role by virtue of the fact that he is probably the only person ever to address the National Right to Life Committee and the National Abortion Rights Action League in the same year. By now all participants were acutely aware of the danger that their years of lobbying and preparation would run aground on the shoals of abortion politics.

THE ADOLESCENT HEALTH, SERVICES AND PREGNANCY PREVENTION AND CARE ACT OF 1978

The "Adolescent Health, Services and Pregnancy Prevention and Care Act of 1978" foundered in the closing period of the Congressional session, as new Congressional attempts to appear to respond to the "tax revolt" signalled by passage of California's ballot proposition 13 overshadowed Carter's and Califano's political problems with the abortion controversy. Then, in a last-minute save, Senator Kennedy tacked the teenage pregnancy language onto DHEW continuing legislation as PL 95-626, Title VI of the Public Health Services Act (92 STAT 3595).

Title VI begins with a restatement of the adolescent pregnancy situation as viewed by most social service providers: that adolescents "are at a high risk of unwanted pregnancy," that 1975 saw 600,000 full-term out of 1,000,000 teen pregnancies, and that pregnancy and childbirth yield "severe adverse health,

social and economic consequences." The Act thus purports to aid in the establishment of improved "coordination, integration, and linkages among existing
programs," to expand the availability of such services, and to "promote innovative, comprehensive, and integrated approaches to the delivery of such
services." The desired result is pregnant adolescents and adolescent parents who
are "productive independent contributors to family and community life."
Persons *under the age of 17* who are *already* pregnant or parents are to receive
principal attention.

Under the terms of the statute, *all* granted programs *must* provide "core
services" which largely entail providing referrals to extramural providers. Pregnancy testing, birth control for those already pregnant, and "primary and preventive" health care must be provided by the granted project (or members of
its "network"). Birth control for nonpregnant clients must only be provided if
"suitable and appropriate" agencies do not already exist in the community to
be served. Screening and treatment for sexually transmitted diseases, pediatric
care, educational and vocational services, adoption arrangements, and "other
appropriate health services" can be covered through referrals to other entities.
Required "core" activities also include many kinds of counseling and informing—"maternity counseling," nutrition information and counseling, sexuality
and family life education, and adoption counseling.

In addition, Title VI *may* (that is, at the discretion of DHEW) cover child
care, consumer and homemaking education, counseling for the adolescent
parent's extended family, transportation to and from caregiving sites, and anything else the Secretary of DHEW decides to cover.

DRAFT PROGRAM REGULATIONS

Draft regulations appeared in the US Federal Register in March 1979. The
proposed regulations seem to "liberal" readers to embody the political diffi-
dence of the legislation itself; in fact, much of the text of the draft regulations
was lifted from the text of PL 95-626 itself.

The proposed regulations reiterated the statute's division of services into
essential "core services" required of grantee agencies and optional "supplementary services" to be funded at the discretion of DHEW. The former included
pregnancy testing, contraceptive services, and pre- and postnatal medical care.
Child care and transportation fell into the "supplemental" category. Grantees
were to develop fee schedules based on the actual cost of services, and to recover
these costs in fee-for-services payments from clients or their parent(s), unless
clients' incomes fell below current Community Services Administration "poverty"
limits. (These limits were $3,140 for a single nonfarm person and $6,200 for a
nonfarm family of four in 1979.) The regulations also followed the statute in

requiring maternity and adoption counseling in granted programs but allowing grantees to limit their involvement with abortion services to informing the pregnant adolescent of the *availability* of abortion counseling. Parental consultation was to be "encouraged" in the pregnant client's decision-making process, unless it be required by state law.

When the proposed regulations were issued, Secretary Califano asked for comments on three areas of concern: the appropriateness of deliberately general regulations as opposed to detailed requirements, the feasibility of requiring applicants to demonstrate explicit agreements with other agencies slated to provide extramural services, and the workability of the fee system.

Before interested parties could prepare their comments on the proposed regulations, a Senate budget hearing on several population issues attracted a major statement on the Adolescent Health, Services, and Pregnancy Prevention and Care Act of 1978 prepared jointly by the American Public Health Association, the American College of Obstetricians and Gynecologists, and the Alan Guttmacher Institute (a Planned Parenthood agency). The statement criticized the administration for its relatively low budget requests for adolescent pregnancy *prevention*:

> A truly comprehensive national program to deal with the problem of adolescent pregnancy would have to include two components: the *prevention* of initial pregnancies among adolescents and supportive services for pregnant adolescents and adolescent parents (Planned Parenthood, 1979a).

Instead of suggesting shifts in the emphasis of the adolescent program itself, the three organizations had decided to link their qualified support of the adolescent bill with demands for higher funding for the existing federal contraception program which most often serves adolescents:

> We stress that an appropriation for the new adolescent pregnancy program *must* be accompanied by an increase in funding for the Family Planning Services and Population Research Act (Title X, Public Health Service Act). There are two major reasons for this. First, as we have already observed, an adolescent pregnancy initiative which focuses entirely on supportive services and ignores prevention is meaningless—and Title X has done more than any other program to prevent unwanted pregnancies among adolescents. Second, the new program will place increased demands on Title X-funded programs since its grantees are required by law to "make maximum use of funds available under Title X of the public Health Service Act" (Planned Parenthood, 1979a).

Planned Parenthood soon submitted lengthy remarks on the proposed adolescent pregnancy program regulations, expressing concerns typical of "liberal" population professionals. The liberals' concerns about the potential for federally funded antiabortion counseling, a source of discord during the earlier Washington meetings between prolife and prochoice activists, surfaced again in an ingenious guise. Prochoice organizations such as Planned Parenthood had been involved in efforts to prevent the use of the informed consent procedure as an antiabortion tactic; now they suggested that informed consent be used in a similar way to force all granted programs to offer genuine pregnancy option counseling:

> In recognition of the importance of childbearing decisions in the lives of all people, and particularly very young persons, we urge you to take steps to ensure that pregnant adolescents fully understand the options available to them and the consequences of their decisions. Regulations for other services provided under DHEW programs require that individuals consenting to certain kinds of medical care be advised of appropriate alternatives to such care, the risks and benefits involved, etc. Young people confronted with an unwanted pregnancy deserve similar protection against any possible coercion. Accordingly, we suggest that the department give serious consideration to developing procedures, such as an informed consent form, to ascertain that adolescents have been provided sufficient information to make a voluntary and informed decision (Planned Parenthood, 1979b).

Planned Parenthood also underscored this concern by suggesting that granted agencies be required to have written referral agreements with agencies whose services they proposed to coordinate, and that

> Grantees should be required to provide assurances (through the submission of formal policies or other means) that pregnant adolescents will be informed of both options regarding the pregnancy: its continuation to term (with the subsequent option of adoption) or its termination. They should also be required to document referrals to the services needed to exercise both options (Planned Parenthood, 1979b).

In short, antiabortion counseling/service agencies such as Birthright, whose services prochoice advocates had been afraid could be funded through the federal program, would not be able to operate without ideological compromise under the Planned Parenthood-suggested regulations.

Another ideological difference between the prochoice and prolife factions appeared in Planned Parenthood's reservations about both the payment and consent portions of the proposed regulations. In essence, Planned Parenthood expressed the general prochoice position on consultation/consent and payment, which is that parental participation in, and approval of, adolescents' reproductive decisions would be nice, but is often impractical. Thus, they recommended that adolescent clients of granted agencies be permitted to declare themselves financially independent of their parents for the purposes of determining fees, and that parental "consultation" never be *required* of young clients even when required by state law (Planned Parenthood, 1979b). In making the latter suggestion, the Planned Parenthood writers were clearly aware of the potential for new legal restrictions on sexually active adolescents inherent in the many recent state parental consent bills proposed and the numerous statutes requiring parental consent now in litigation.

FINAL PROGRAM REGULATIONS

Many of the "liberal" platform planks were included in the final regulations which were published in the Federal Register in June 1979. The fee system now must be structured to permit adolescent clients to act independently of their families for the purposes of obtaining funded services. Parental consultation is still "encouraged," but not required even if state law requires it. Information, education, counseling, and referral services are to be provided essentially free of charge, permitting entry-type services to be provided in as accessible a fashion as possible. Applicants are not *required* to prove preexisting arrangements with referral agencies, but priority in granting is to be given to applicants who do provide such proof. The final regulations also recognize the independence of adolescent clients by explicitly requiring that records be held confidential. Standards for each service, to be based on Titles V and X of the Public Health Services Act, were left to the department's program guidelines.

As the final regulations reached concerned agencies, the climate at DHEW was somewhat changed by the resignation of Secretary Joseph Califano and the confirmation of Patricia Roberts Harris as his successor. During Senate confirmation hearings in July 1979, Harris indicated attitudes toward abortion far more liberal than those of her predecessor Califano. Noting that she agreed with Surgeon General Julius Richmond that the legalization of abortions had contributed to a decrease in rates of morbidity and mortality due to illegal abortions, Harris declared that she would have "no problem, in fact quite the contrary" in supporting the provision of information about the abortion alternative to adolescent pregnancies throughout the new adolescent pregnancy program her department was to administer. Planned Parenthood's Washington Memo expressed a general "liberal" hope that Harris's accession would protect them from the service limitations they had feared at the hands of the antiabortion Califano:

Judging from Mrs. Harris' remark that "so long that this [abortion] is a protected right . . . information is almost a duty," it would seem that DHEW policy may be expected to emphasize the right of individuals to receive information about all pregnancy options. . . Prochoice supporters should take heart at Mrs. Harris' personal views on public funding of abortions—certainly a far cry from former Secretary Califano's unequivocal opposition. However, given Mrs. Harris' pledge to obey the law and the law as currently written, what impact her personal views can and will have on either DHEW policy or the availability of Medicaid funds to provide abortions for low-income women remains to be seen (Planned Parenthood, 1979c).

PROGRAM FUNDING

It now remained to secure funding for the program. The Carter administration requested $7 million in "start up" funds for the first year of the program, to be followed by $60 million in fiscal year (FY) 1980. This request applied to supplemental funds to be expended during the remainder of FY 1979 (that is the federal fiscal year, which starts October 1). When the House and Senate completed their separate budget deliberations, the Senate recommended $1 million in startup funds for the adolescent program for the remainder of FY 1979; the members of the House felt that the entire program could wait until FY 1980 to begin. Thus, requests for proposals reached potential program applicants before funding was secured, and some local groups negotiated linkages and cooperative plans with a feeling of futility.

When the differing House and Senate recommendations on funding for family planning and the adolescent pregnancy program reached a conference committee, the Senate conferees expressed their membership's feeling that family planning should be a high health care funding priority in the FY 1979 supplementary budget, while House conferees continued to oppose any further health care funds for the fiscal year. When the conference committee finally reported its compromise version of the supplementary budget, $1 million was listed for start up office-staffing monies. Family planning services received no supplementary funds, although population research programs gained another $7.5 million.

Meanwhile, segments of both houses of Congress were working on the FY 1980 budget. Population program advocates were pleased (albeit surprised) to see both Senate and House Labor/HEW appropriations subcommittees recommending funding levels for Title X above those of the previous year. As expected on all sides, much of the Congress's attention to population matters was focused on the annual struggle over the antiabortion Hyde Amendment to the Medicaid portion of the Labor/HEW budget. Ironically, the tense temper of Congress over the Hyde Amendment probably led to higher funding levels for family planning; when the Title X budget passed the House and Senate in July, Title X received $165 million, a $30 million increase over the previous year's allocation. In fact, when the Hyde amendment smoke cleared the following October, Title X was the *only* major social service program granted an increase over Administration requests, and the Title X appropriation was undisputed in Congress for the first time in the ten years of its existence.

When the Senate Appropriations Committee issued its FY 1979 supplemental budget report, its $1 million recommendation for the adolescent pregnancy program was accompanied by language which indicated that Congressional support of the program was still complicated by disagreements over its vulnerability to manipulation by DHEW itself or by politically motivated grantees. The supplementary item included a requirement that "all facets of the so-called prolife and prochoice factions" be represented on Office of Adolescent Pregnancy Programs staff and advisory bodies, and that "a report be given to the Committee prior to any grant or contract being let, specifying how each contract will result in the complete review of all options open to the pregnant adolescent." This provision was removed, however, at the behest of prolife Senator Richard Schweiker.

As FY 1980 appropriations were developed in each house of Congress, the residues of earlier legislative concerns remained. The House only appropriated one quarter of the Administration's requested amount for the adolescent pregnancy program, indicating its concern with the role of prevention in the new program by tying this smaller appropriation to a larger allocation for Title X family planning funds. The text of the Senate's $20 million appropriation for 1980 called for clarification of DHEW's "preparedness for program implementation" through submission of a closely defined report:

> Describing plans for program administration, including criteria and priorities established for making grant awards, program evaluation plans, plans to issue final regulations which clarify the legislation and other issues relevant to the management of a sound program.

In the end, the appropriation for the Adolescent Health, Services, Pregnancy Prevention and Care Act settled out at $17.5 million, typically splitting the difference between the House and Senate figures.

FIRST-PHASE GRANTS

The first phase of the program awarded grants to four programs for a total of $740,000 of the $1 million in FY 1980 start up funds; the granted programs were scheduled to begin operations in spring 1980. The kind of project chosen by DHEW in the first phase suggests that it has followed its own regulations and guidelines in selecting community-based projects with preexisting coordination of agency services. DHEW has also chosen to view its granting powers in terms of "pilot" or "seed money" models; the new programs are to receive funds for five years, but will suffer a ten percent decline in funds (and thus a larger relative decline) each year.

THE FUTURE OF SERVICES TO CHILDBEARING ADOLESCENTS

Services for childbearing adolescents have been facilitated and constrained by the crosscurrents described in the aforementioned legislative history: differing views of sexual morality, attitudes toward abortion, and ideas about the role of public programs in reinforcing normative behavior have molded both lobbying and legislative behavior in response to the problems of childbearing adolescents. Although the Adolescent Health, Service, Pregnancy Prevention and Care Act entailed funding projections over several years, the program is vulnerable to limitations, both fiscal and operational, at the hands of Congress. The adolescent health services system as a whole is also open to the effect of broad social forces beyond its control.

Forces which will act to constrain the provision of services to childbearing adolescents can be divided arbitrarily into three types for heuristic purposes: changes in demand, limits on funding, and restraints on services offered.

CHANGES IN DEMAND

Although the cluster of causes of increased adolescent childbearing to which one subscribes depends on political and cultural orientations, most providers agree that broad socioeconomic factors have more effect on service demand than do the inroads of contraceptive programs. If fiscal and cultural conservatism led to a reduction in the availability of sexuality education and contraception, the increase in adolescent pregnancies would probably be relatively small and some of that increase would be absorbed by abortions. Significant changes in the legal or financial basis for adolescent access to abortion would also affect demand for childbearing services, but the magnitude of this effect is hard to calculate in the absence of any historical precedent. Absence of precedent has also made it difficult for observers to clarify the relationship between contraceptive practice and abortion utilization for adolescents—that is, does the availability of abortion reduce the use of contraception among adolescents or is abortion a last resort, outside the contraception decision entirely? In sum, it is as unreliable to fear a great increase in adolescent childbearing because of changes in contraception and abortion as it is to assume that the sudden adoption of an ideal national contraception system would significantly reduce the adolescent pregnancy rate.

National and regional economic conditions, however, seem to have a clearer or more calculable effect on adolescent childbearing rates. Providers suggest that local unemployment and underemployment contribute to an atmosphere in which adolescents perceive limited life chances, and girls, already disadvantaged by pervasive sexism at the workplace, may see (at least unconsciously) some advantage in establishing independent households rather than in remaining in financially taxed parental homes. The growing incidence of single parent households has reduced the stigma which led adolescent childbearers to seek adoption for their infants in the past, even if the social services available to single parents have not improved the desperate situation in which many will find themselves. Thus, current socioeconomic conditions can only be expected to contribute to *increased* demand for services to adolescent parents.

FUNDING

Political forces which led to broad Republican electoral gains in the 1980 elections are now analytically separated into two components by political pundits: the "traditional" conservatism of the Republic Party as a whole, and the "New Right" conservatism which finds its focus in matters of personal morality, school policy, and the like. The electoral success of both "conservative" forces in the 1970s can be expected to exert a restraining influence on public funding for new and existing services to childbearing adolescents. "Traditional" conservatism among voters and legislators will have the effect of reducing absolute funding levels and abolishing social service programs of many kinds. "New Right" conservatism can be expected to make even reduced funding for contraceptive care and, particularly, abortion services nearly impossible to secure. If, as prochoice activists have often claimed, there is a substantial component of punitiveness toward nonmarital sexual activity in political opposition to abortion, this attitude will further endanger programs for childbearing adolescents if they are seen as encouraging or rewarding deviant sexual behavior. Since day care programs are often the target of "pro-family" attempts to limit professional intervention in family processes, it will probably continue to be difficult to provide the day care services often regarded as crucial to comprehensive adolescent parent programs. The United States is already years behind Europe in institutionalizing supports for working parents and/or single parents; there is nothing to suggest that the "move to the right" of the 1970s and 1980s will do anything to accelerate the social acceptance of widespread day care. There is a particular aversion among "New Right" conservatives to infant day care; this very expensive service is regarded by many advocates of comprehensive adolescent parent programs as a critical contributor to improving young parents' educational and employment prospects.

SERVICES

Aside from already-noted constraints through funding processes on abortion, childcare, and even contraception, federal and state legislators have shown a continued desire to do two things which would limit the services available to pregnant adolescents: to limit the availability of abortion to the maximum extent possible, and to impose parental notification, consultation, or consent requirements on agencies treating adolescents. Battles among prolife and prochoice lobbyists interested in adolescent pregnancy programs over the status of abortion counseling indicate a gap in perceptions of the parameters of adequate psychological counseling since each group has a different view of the "correct" or "mature" adolescent pregnancy decision. Prochoice professionals tend to assume that an effective counseling intervention will tend to lead to abortion of the nonmarital pregnancy, while prolife professionals suspect parental coercion or counseling bias if the counselee chooses not to carry her pregnancy to term. For prochoice providers and legislators alike, publicly funded services that prohibit any mention of the availability of abortion to the counselee are irresponsibly truncated. For the prolife provider or legislator, programs that permit or mandate counseling without mention of the possibility of abortion exert a desirable philosophical counterthrust to the "abortion-mindedness" of society as a whole. Legislators who take the latter position can be expected to regulate the provision of abortion counseling-cum-provision of services as far as the courts will permit. These regulations have already included elaborate informed consent procedures involving discussions of fetal development, heartbeat, brainwaves, etc. and waiting periods between the counseling session and performance of the abortion. Prochoice providers regard such restrictions as unnecessary and punitive additions to the trauma of the abortion experience. Their profile counterparts regard legally imposed informed consent procedures as valuable opportunities for aborting patients to understand the true nature of abortion and to make final decisions outside the atmosphere of clinics devoted to the performance of abortions.

Parental consent issues have been argued in court periodically for the last several years. The most famous case, initially known as Baird v. Bellotti, arose when the Massachusetts legislature attempted to require that minors obtain their parents' permission before undergoing abortions in the state. Baird, a provider, has successfully argued that such a law unconstitutionally limits adolescents' access to abortions, but some legal observers expect that when the issue reaches the Supreme Court it may move to mandate some kind of parental consultation without veto power. Again, prochoice providers fear that comprehensive services to adolescents will be hampered by their clients' fears of parental disapproval such that adolescents will fail to seek professional services until their pregnancies are too far advanced to forestall full-term childbirth. If such parental permission statutes spread to other adolescent health services (contraception, treatment of sexually transmitted diseases, and general sexuality counseling), comprehensive services would be faced with complex problems of permission, notification, and the practical loss of provider/client confidentiality.

PROSPECTS

If the increasing fiscal/moral conservatism of electorates and legislators has the effects outlined above, providers are actually presented with a model of maximum remaining service effectiveness in the "linkage" component of the Adolescent Health, Services, Pregnancy Prevention and Care Act itself. Existing large institutional providers—hospitals, long-term clinics, schools, and large voluntary organizations—can best weather shifts in the levels and emphases of public funding because the adolescent portions of their programs represent small proportions of their total operating budgets. Although such linked services are easier to establish in relatively compact urban areas, necessity may force even rural areas to meet adolescent childbearers' needs through rationally linked existing medical, education, child care, and employment services. Medical and educational services, of course, are more immune to changes in public support than are child care and employment services unless these exist within the framework of public education.

Limitations on providing abortions and contraception cannot be bypassed through linkages and the use of older institutions, of course. Inevitably, the burden of provision will fall on large voluntary entities such as Planned Parenthood and through them on private donors committed to continued levels of contraceptive and abortion care. Prochoice organizations may find that they need to shift their emphasis from political and legal action to simple underwriting of services.

Perhaps the most important lesson of the legislative history of the Adolescent Health, Services, Pregnancy Prevention and Care Act is that the difficult political climate surrounding all issues of sexuality and reproduction can best be weathered by a coalition of prolife and prochoice parties. Such coalitions are difficult to forge because of the differences in cultural meanings between the two kinds of groups; however, the era of large grants to liberal social service organizations may have passed, and those interested in continuity of services must be prepared to swallow jurisdictional and ideological differences.

SUMMARY

A legislative history of the Adolescent Health, Services and Pregnancy Prevention and Care Act of 1978 is outlined. The Act resulted from pressure on President Jimmy Carter to provide the alternatives to abortion he espoused during the 1976 presidential campaign, the efforts of a prolife/prochoice lobbying coalition in Washington, and the efforts of researchers for DHEW Secretary Califano. After quiet disagreement with the administration text because of its vagueness and the ambiguity of the position of abortion counseling and provision services, the bill was passed as part of the Public Health Services Act in 1978. The required federal regulations for implementation of mandated programs were issued in draft form and revised in response to provider and political group pressure and suggestions. Pilot programs were granted funds after initial funding was approved by Congress in 1979. Prospects for continued funding, demand on services, and limitation on the nature of services provided through such programs are discussed, suggesting that the moral and fiscal conservatism which characterizes recent voter behavior and recently elected candidates may mean decreased funding and increased legal limitations on services (especially abortions) without corresponding reductions in demand through reduction in the adolescent childbearing and childkeeping rate.

ADDENDUM

Several political developments have altered the landscape of programs for sexually active and childbearing adolescents since this chapter was written. In short, "New Right" and Reagan Administration forces have combined to constrain adolescents' access to contraceptive and abortion services, and opposing forces have countered with legal and legislative efforts of their own.

When Title X came up for reauthorization in 1981 opponents of contraceptive services for adolescents attempted to combine those services with other medical programs in a more easily attacked block grant. Congressional supporters of Title X managed to maintain its status as a categorical program and to preserve adequate funding levels. At the same time, however, Sen. Jeremiah Denton's (R-Ala.) Adolescent Family Life Act (familiarly known as the "chastity bill" for its emphasis on discouraging adolescent sexual activity) became Title Xb of the Public Health Services Act (42 USC 300). The Office of Adolescent Pregnancy Programs was disbanded and all Federal funds for childbearing adolescents came to be administered through the new Office of Adolescent Family Life Programs. Since then, activity surrounding Federal involvement in adolescent childbearing has reflected conservatives' realization that administrative measures of control are easier to achieve than are legislative victories. From its inception, the OAFLP has been headed by Marjory Mecklenburg, antiabortion veteran of the Washington coalition responsible for urging Federal involvement in adolescent childbearing in the first place (see "The Prolife/Prochoice Coalition," p. 202) (Planned Parenthood, 1983a).

In January, 1983, outgoing Secretary of Health and Human Services Richard Schweiker moved Titles X and Xb out of the Bureau of Health Care Delivery and Assistance of the Public Health Service, where they had been administered by public health professionals, into a new Office of Family Planning in the Office of Population Affairs under the Assistant Secretary for Health Affairs, a political appointee. Both programs are now under the supervision of the new Deputy Assistant Secretary for Population Affairs Marjory Mecklenburg, who has been charged with "assuring consistency between the Title X and Title Xb programs (Planned Parenthood, 1983a). At this juncture (Fall, 1983), Title Xb grantees are required to obtain parental consent to the provision of services to their minor clients, unless, apparently, parents seem inclined to counsel abortion. The placement of clients' babies for adoption is to be encouraged, as adolescent sexual activity is to be discouraged. Information about abortion is not to be provided in granted programs, and referrals to family agencies require special parental consent procedures and verification (Planned Parenthood, 1983b).

Administration attempts to place similar restrictions on Title X programs through Departmental regulations mechanisms have been rebuffed by the Federal courts, leaving adolescents' access to confidential contraceptive services and advice intact for the moment (Planned Parenthood, 1983b). A Government Accounting Office audit of Title X programs has also failed to turn up any evidence of the abortion activities and political activism of which grantees have long been accused by their opponents (Planned Parenthood, 1983a).

Title Xb programs were budgeted at approximately $13 million for fiscal year 1983. Title X received $124 million for the same period. These figures reflect neither their advocates' requests nor their detractors' suggested cuts.

REFERENCES

Alan Guttmacher Institute. 1976. *11 Million Teenagers.* New York: Planned Parenthood Federation of America.
Crittenden Hastings House. 1978. *1978 Annual Report.* Boston: Crittenden Hastings House.
Ordway v. Hargraves. 1971. 323 F. Supp. @ 1155.
Planned Parenthood-World Population. 1979a. *Washington Memo,* W-6 (April 6):2.
Planned Parenthood-World Population. 1979b. *Washington Memo,* W-7 (April 7):2.

Planned Parenthood-World Population. 1979c. *Washington Memo,* W-13 (September 14):2.
Planned Parenthood-World Population. 1983a. *Washington Memo,* W-1 (January 19):1, 2.
Planned Parenthood-World Population. 1983b. *Washington Memo,* W-13 (July 27):1.
U.S. Congress. Senate Committee on Human Resources. *Adolescent Pregnancy Hearings.* June 28, 1978a. MC 78-26766 LC 78-603248.
U.S. Congress. Senate Committee on Human Resources. *Adolescent Pregnancy Hearings.* July 24, 1978b. MC 78-26815 LC 78-603215.
U.S. Federal Register. March 12, 1979, 44:49.
U.S. Federal Register. July 23, 1979, 44:142.
Zero Population Growth. 1978. *ZPG National Reporter* 10(4):7.

13

The Family Context
of Adolescent Parenting

THEODORA OOMS

Professionals and policy makers alike have neglected the primary social context in which teenage pregnancy and parenthood takes place, namely, the family context. Most teenagers are living with their families when they initiate sexual activity and when pregnancy occurs. And at least 80 percent of the unmarried teenage women who give birth remain living with their families. Although teenagers are undoubtedly much influenced by their peers and the media, it is their families who are their primary source of long-term caring and support. The health, educational, and social service programs developed to help teenage mothers and their babies have largely ignored the others affected by teenage parenthood. There has been some recognition of the role of the teenage male in teen sex and pregnancy and of the needs of teenage fathers. But what of the role of parents in teenage sexual behavior? And how are they—as well as brothers, sisters, grandparents, and other family members—affected by adolescent parenthood?

The short answer to these questions is that we do not know very much and we need to know more. Research has been influenced by an ethos of individualism; the focus and training have been to study individuals, often in laboratory or medical settings away from the contexts in which they live and separate from their relationships with the significant people in their lives (Bronfenbrenner, 1979). Only recently have researchers and clinicians come to realize that it is important to understand individuals in their different contexts (Minuchin and Fishman, 1981) and that such an approach has important clinical and policy implications. This chapter will review what is known about the

217

family context of teenage pregnancy and parenthood and will speculate briefly on why the family's role has been so neglected. It will then suggest that we know enough to recommend that policy makers and professionals need to take account of the powerful role and resources of families if they want their programs and services to be effective.

In her review of the research literature about the role of the family of origin in teenage sexual behavior, Fox (1981) asked whether certain kinds of family structure, characteristics, or patterns of communication appear to be associated with teenage sexual activity or early pregnancy. Despite the small amount of research on these questions and the fact that most of the samples were of college students, certain conclusions emerged clearly. There is little direct communication about sex between parents and children, and when it does occur it is most often between mother and daughter. (There are many avenues of *indirect* communication, for example, modelling of sex roles and attitudes which need more exploration.) While parents may never have been the source of accurate or complete information about the facts of sex, previous generations of parents probably provided a clearer set of values, attitudes, and expectations about sexual behavior. Today's changing sexual standards make it harder for parents to be consistent in what they think and believe; thus, they adopt an "ostrich attitude" towards their teenagers' sexual behavior and provide unclear messages and guidance (Fox, 1981; Furstenberg, 1981).

A most important finding that Fox (1981) highlights in her review is that when parents (usually the mother) communicate openly and explicitly with their children about sex, *irrespective of the content of this discussion*, this communication seems to delay the start of sexual activity. Furthermore, once sex is initiated, explicit communication seems to be associated with more effective use of contraceptives. There are many implications of this finding for family involvement in preventive programs of sex education and contraceptive counseling (Ooms, 1981). Fox (1981) and Furstenberg (1981) both suggested that parents play a significant role when an adolescent is faced with decisions about pregnancy. This is underscored in research by Rosen and Benson (1979) in a rural area of Michigan, which illustrates the influence, even in an indirect form, that parents have on pregnant teenagers' decision whether to abort or not. They found that three quarters of those pregnant teenagers who chose abortion but did not tell their parents indicated that fear of hurting their parents, or of their parents' anger if told about the pregnancy, influenced their decision to abort.

Various family developmental issues and crises may contribute unconsciously to a teenager's becoming pregnant, or at least to her decision to keep rather than to abort her baby. In the days of more shotgun marriages, pregnancy was clearly a route that some girls followed to get out of a troubled home setting. Now, it may more often be a way of being welcomed back into the bosom of the family, and receiving a greater degree of attention and higher status within the family (Furstenberg, 1981). Other family events or crises may also be linked with an adolescent pregnancy, such as her mother's having a surprise menopausal baby, depression upon facing the loss of her own reproductive capacities, or the prospect of an empty nest. Pregnancy can also involve a reaction to a recent loss such as major surgery to the girl, the boyfriend going to jail, or the death of a father or close relative (Sugar, personal communication, 1981, 1982).

Fox's (1981) review of the literature supports Furstenberg's (1976) research findings that once a teenager decides to go ahead with pregnancy her family plays an important role in her various life decisions: whether to keep the baby or give it up, whether to marry, where to live, who will care for the baby, and whether to go back to school. Her family's views about the baby's father are often the controlling factor in the extent to which he is allowed to see his baby or otherwise stay involved. Furstenberg reported that 70 to 80 percent of the teenage mothers lived with their parents through pregnancy and the first months of the baby's life, and the majority stayed on for several years after. Although his sample predominantly included low income blacks, data from other small studies suggest this living pattern may be consistent for whites and Hispanics also (see Chapter 6, this volume, for variation among Hispanics). In addition to housing, family members provide various kinds of practical and psychological support—child care in particular. Furthermore, adolescent mothers who received assistance from their families and remained living with them were more likely to return to school and less likely to receive long-term welfare assistance than teen parents who married and/or moved away from their parents' home. When an adolescent brings her baby home other members of her family may have their own lives affected in quite direct ways: the baby's grandmother may quit her job, there may be more harmony or more strife between the grandparents, a young uncle may feel competitive and displaced in the family's affections, a young aunt may even become pregnant herself (Furstenberg, 1981). The positive impact of family support on the welfare of a teenage mother and her child is emerging in a number of ongoing studies, reviewed in an article by Baldwin and Cain (1980).

In exploring the impact of the teenage mother and her child on the other family members in a small pilot study, Furstenberg (1981) described some of the roles family members play in accomodating to the event. He identified a variety of tasks that need to be accomplished by the family as a system when a teenager has a baby. Primary among these is the decision about who should be involved in caring for the child. Although there are a variety of arrangements, varying from those carefully planned to those quite haphazard, some kind of multiple caretaking is the norm in these families, and siblings play an important role. Consequently, the adolescent mother's status is often somewhat ambiguous.

Furstenberg speculated that arrangements that are relatively harmonious in the first months of a "honeymoon period" after the birth may become the subject of considerable conflict as the baby becomes more difficult to cope with and as the adolescent mother is expected to assume increasing responsibility. Furstenberg's study raises many family-related questions of which a program serving adolescents should be aware.

This new research evidence documenting the involvement of families in adolescent sexual behavior and its consequences is persuasive since it corresponds to many personal clinical experiences and poignant expressions in literature and the media. But how is it that until quite recently we viewed the adolescent girl as the sole target for our prevention and treatment efforts?

A number of factors accounted in part for this narrow focus. Among these were the attitudes towards illegitimacy which led pregnant young white women to search for help secretly or far from home, and the condemnation of her community, which accounted for the fact that most white babies born out of wedlock were given up for adoption. A second reason was that in the 1950s and 1960s it was medical leadership which brought to the public's attention the health risks incurred by premature pregnancy and advocated improved health care for pregnant teenagers and their infants. Third, these decades also saw the emergence of the movement to give women control over their own bodies through controlling fertility. Adolescent women were considered by many to have the same rights in these respects as adult women, and to be entitled to the same rules of confidentiality and privacy.

This latter theme may account for the continuing resistance on the part of many professionals, policy makers, and the public to adopt a family-oriented approach to teenage sexuality and for the controversy over issues of parental notification and consent.

As a society we are confused about the status of adolescents in general and their rights and responsibilities. Nowhere is this more true than with regard to their sexual behavior. Sexual maturity defines new boundaries between parent and child. When the adolescent engages in sexual activity, perhaps more than any other activity it symbolizes the impending separation from parents. Such physical maturity and its acting out is coming at earlier and earlier ages, ironically when the other symbols of adulthood (completing education and getting a job) for many are becoming increasingly delayed.

Pregnancy dramatically signals to the family and world outside that, in one dimension at least, adult status has been achieved. Paradoxically, this same pregnancy, if continued usually thrusts the teenage girl and sometimes her partner into renewed dependence on parents and other adults (doctors, counselors, etc.). Now that marriage is rarely chosen as a solution to unwed pregnancy, it is less clear that pregnancy is a step towards independence. Indeed, for a few, becoming pregnant may be a way back into the family or a way of acquiring greater status within the family, as Furstenberg (1981) reported.

The family perspective is not easy for professionals working with adolescents; whether teacher, youth leader, family planning counselor or doctor, if an advocate for the student/client/patient, the tendency is to think in terms of adolescent rights and needs and to lose sight of the rights, needs, and responsibilities of other family members. Health care professionals in particular have a very difficult task when providing sex-related medical care to young persons. They are concerned about respecting the adolescent's confidentiality and ensuring easy access to needed health services. They must make difficult judgments about a teenager's psychological and moral maturity, and her capacity to make informed decisions (Hofmann and Moore, 1982). In addition, theories about the extent to which adolescents engaging in sex and becoming pregnant are acting out unconscious conflicts with pathology-producing parents have a long history (Young, 1954) and may still be influencing professional attitudes toward the parents of teenage clients. Thus, we have arrived at the situation where most professional associations assert the right of a minor adolescent to seek and obtain sex-related health care without parental notification and consent (Pilpel and Wechsler, 1971), although the same adolescent may need parental consent for other areas of health care (minor surgery or a blood test) or in other spheres of life (for example, to obtain a learner's license or get employment). Most state laws have recognized this right through a variety of emancipation or mature minor statutes; the US Supreme Court has denied parents the right to consent (or veto) with regard to contraceptive care and abortion, but has left the issue of parental notice somewhat ambiguous (Ooms, 1981; Gothard, 1980).

This consensus among professionals is challenged by more conservative and traditional members of the public—and the politicians who represent their views—as a position that undermines parental authority and responsibilities and is ultimately antifamily. Legislation introduced in the US Congress in 1981, and in several state legislatures, seeks to assert the rights of parents in sex-related health care. This controversy—fully discussed elsewhere (Ooms, 1981)—exemplifies in extreme fashion the fact that the design of many policies and programs, and the attitude and training of most staff, are seldom oriented towards involving the adolescent's family when providing sex-related health services.

The confusion and ambivalence with regard to helping the sexually active adolescent is also reflected in policies and programs which aim to meet the needs of the adolescent parent. For example, a major federal source of financial assistance to teenage parents—the Aid to Families with Dependent Children (AFDC) program—is in some states only available to teenage mothers who leave their parental home. In some other states, the teenager's *baby* is eligible for AFDC even if the teenager is living with her parents who have sufficient income, are not themselves receiving welfare, and are supporting their daughter. Thus, her baby becomes an independent source of income for the adolescent mother. Paradoxically, the grandparents who may in fact be sharing much of the cost and day-to-day responsibility of caring for their grandchild have no legal rights or responsibilities toward their grandchild.

Policy concerning the father is also quite confused. The unmarried father has in general no rights, even to be consulted about the pregnancy or the fate of the child. And yet the federal government's Child Support Enforcement Program pursues a vigorous policy of establishing paternity for an unmarried father (through blood tests) in order to attempt to collect child support from him either now or in the future when he has some income. We have little hard data on the extent to which teen fathers are in fact identified in this program; however, there is no doubt that the fear of their partner's being forced to admit paternity keeps many teenage girls from admitting that they know who the father is, with the result that many teenage fathers keep a very low profile, even though there is increasing evidence that they are often interested in the baby and in being helpful (see Chapter 5, this volume). We have to question then whether present policy is designed to encourage male responsibility and involvement or whether it does not have the opposite effect.

At the level of actual programs for teenage parents, a number of important questions are suggested by a family perspective. Since the evidence points to the strong influence (whether positive or negative) of her family, how do agency staff assess the family situation of their teenage client? As mentioned, the traditional approach has been to regard the teen parent as an autonomous individual. An informal survey reported by Forbush and Maciocha (1981) confirms that, although there are a few notable exceptions, most adolescent parent programs do *not* involve the teenager's family. But can one rely on just the teenager herself for an account of the kinds of assistance her family is willing to provide her? Is it appropriate to provide only her with medical advice and parenting education when she may indeed not be the primary caretaker, or when her mother or some other adult member believes, because of their particular cultural and educational background, in caring for the baby in ways that the clinic staff think are wrong or misguided? Should the teen parent be supported in her desire to get away from the conflict and arguments with her mother about caring for the baby, and encouraged to live independently? Or would it be more realistic to attempt to mediate the difficulties and recognize her need to continue to be dependent? Should the relationship with the baby's father and his family be encouraged or discouraged? Should the client's siblings be involved in the hope that they may avoid repeating her early pregnancy experience? These are just a few of the questions that program staff need to ask themselves.

If adolescent parenthood is viewed from a family perspective, what implications does this have for programs and policies? There is a good deal of current rhetoric about the need for more family involvement programs (see particularly the language in the new Title XX, of the Public Health Service Act of 1981 providing further funding for Adolescent Family Life Demonstration Projects). Yet it has not been clear just what increased family involvement means in practice.

There are at least two levels at which families can be "involved": the involvement of families whose adolescents obtain services and the more general involvement of families from the wider community whose teenagers may or may not be potential clients of the agency.

The following are a few suggested guidelines for serving adolescent parents in their family context. They include assessing the level and nature of family support and resources, and designing services that where possible complement and build upon the family's own resources rather than substituting or competing with them.

During the intake process and later as well, staff should collect information about the teenager's family situation: to what extent the families (hers and/or her partner's) are able to provide shelter, economic assistance, and infant care; to what extent other family members share in the care of the baby; and whether the sharing of responsibilities creates much stress and conflict or is relatively harmonious. This kind of information is best obtained not only from the adolescents but also from other family members, who should be invited to join in the interviews. The teenager's parents, grandparents, siblings, and close friends should all be considered as potential sources of information, support, and help in planning what the agency's own role and services should be.

Such an assessment of the client's family context is best done in a home visit—yet agency policies, neighborhood factors, and reimbursement practices tend to discourage such visits which years ago were considered routine in many social agencies. Such interviews with the teenager and other family members require special skills and training for those whose only experience is working with individuals and who do not know how to help a family negotiate and work out their own problems. It is also important that staff be able to assess when a family situation is so disorganized, chaotic, or in such turmoil that specially trained help or referral to agencies more experienced in therapy and preventive work with families is needed.

Prenatal, obstetric, and postnatal programs (including well baby and pediatric clinics) must be flexible about which significant family members should be encouraged to accompany the teenage girl to her appointments and join her in discussions with medical personnel. This support is also critical during her labor (and delivery) and her stay in the maternity ward. Some programs are now willing to involve the teenage father and/or her mother, sister, aunt, or even a friend. Unfortunately, many still do not. Such practices are essential for the adolescent to obtain support, and may be critical in ensuring that medical advice and recommendations are followed through regarding her own care or that of her child. They may lead to a discovery that the clinic's advice to the young parent and her own mother's are in conflict or that the new grandmother and mother have not yet worked out an acceptable way of sharing child care responsibilities. The meetings may help the grandmother to be a more effective teacher for her daughter.

In addressing the adolescent's plans for the future, the service program needs to be aware of her family context. The issues of completing school or getting training or a job in order to avoid long-term dependency on public assistance—which has been the future of many teenage mothers—need to be discussed. An important corollary is to explore motivation for successful contraception to prevent another pregnancy following too rapidly on the first. These issues and the need for follow-up services and referral must be raised with the teenager herself and with the significant others in her family. Harper (1981) provides powerful descriptive evidence of the sometimes subtle and sometimes quite direct ways in which family members (including in one instance brothers) resist and counteract efforts of the young mother to return to school or get a job and become more independent. Exploring plans for the future must also involve whoever in her family has the most influence upon the adolescent mother to ensure that the program's goals and efforts are not working at cross purposes with those of the family. At times, certainly, a deliberate decision may be made to counter the family's influence and to support the autonomy of the adolescent; however, it is still necessary to assess the strength and direction of the family's influence.

There are indeed times when a pregnant adolescent or adolescent parent is seriously estranged from her family (Perlman, 1980). Information in a client's case record (if, for example, she is referred from some other social service agency) may alert the agency to the adolescent for whom no family resources or support are available. (Such information should emerge from the intake process and attempts to assess the family situation.) The adolescent may be fleeing from a home with serious abuse, alcoholism, or mental illness. She may be a product of the foster care system.

It is important to explore with the client whether extended family or other adult friends in the community are a possible resource to her. If none are available, then serious consideration must be given to identifying some community persons or organizations who may serve as surrogate families, ombudsmen, or role models to the young parent. They can serve a purpose that no formal program or agency counselor can fulfill (see Chapter 11, this volume).

Family involvement does not mean that adolescent parent programs need to transform themselves into family service agencies, meeting all the needs of everyone in the teenage parent's family. But in meeting the teen's needs, they must at least recognize what other needs exist within the family. It may happen that an agency decides, as some have, to design special services for other family members—such as a grandmothers' discussion group or employment counseling for teenage fathers—or to encourage younger siblings to come in for sex education or family planning services. A family perspective may lead to the recognition that helping the teenage mother's *mother* get a job, needed health care, or into alcoholism treatment is the most effective way of helping the teenager with her current stressful situation of continual conflict with her mother. In general, the staff will need to be trained to refer the other family members to appropriate services elsewhere.

There are administrative and professional barriers that can make it very difficult to implement a family-oriented approach. For example, agencies are often not reimbursed by third party payers for services that are not directly given to the individual client or patient. Working with families in the short run may take more time (for example, making home visits) and programs that depend on high client-staff ratios may not be able to adjust. Perhaps the most important barrier, as Furstenberg et al (1981) pointed out (when describing a program that involves the kinship system in family planning services), is that health and social service personnel need considerable reorienting of their role toward the adolescent *and* her family. Training in the skills of assessing family functioning, in interviewing several members of a family together, and especially in being able to mediate family disagreements and conflicts may all be needed. The professional may need to think of him or herself not as a provider of information, counseling, and advice or treatment to the teenage clients but rather as a facilitator, enabler, trainer, or consultant to teenagers and their entire family.

As mentioned earlier, another level of family involvement is that of the community in general. This helps agencies and clinics to be more sensitive to the cultural patterns of the community and to reflect the family perspective more adequately in their policies and practices.

Agencies should actively seek to involve parents, adolescents, and other family members in the community to serve as members of boards and advisory and planning committees, as volunteers, or as paid paraprofessional staff. Efforts should be made to obtain such community input on issues of program design and policy, particularly when program staff are from a different socioeconomic, racial, or ethnic background than their clientele. This kind of community and consumer input is rare in services to adolescents, although it has been a required element in programs for other age groups such as Head Start. Another way of obtaining feedback is to hold regular discussion meetings with groups of teenage clients and/or their parents to ask for suggestions of ways to improve agency practices.

Service programs should make the community which provides their private or public funding aware of the families they serve, and that they attempt to complement, not replace, a teen's family and their resources. They should collect information on family backgrounds and on the kind and degree of assistance adolescents receive from their families in order to assess client needs, plan program services to meet these needs, and to try to account for any differences in outcome.

Directions suggested above for a family approach to adolescent parent programs have been and are being tried out somewhere; for the most part they have yet to be fully evaluated. Experience from other fields of service delivery, such as mental health where family therapy has been well-evaluated, suggests that it is an approach that not only makes good clinical sense but may also make good economic sense. If the nature and degree of services to the teen parent are built upon a careful assessment of the resources available to her from her own family and community, there is less likely to be duplication of service or undercutting of program efforts. Further, viewing her family as partners provides the professional agency with more leverage and reinforcement of its own efforts. And finally, outreach to the family is more likely to distinguish those adolescents whose family situations are so fragile, nonexistent, or hostile that they need special degrees of support to prevent the isolation and despair that leads to inadequate parenting and neglect.

SUMMARY

This chapter has argued that there are sound social, scientific, and clinical reasons for approaching the problems of adolescent parenthood from a family perspective. Redesigning programs to build on, and supplement, families' own resources and efforts—and only substitute for families when absolutely necessary—may well be the most effective and efficient way to help adolescents and their infants.

REFERENCES

Adolescent Family Life Demonstration Projects, 1981. *Title XX Public Health Service Act.* Incorporated in U.S. Budget Reconciliation Act, HR 3982, sec. 955.
Baldwin, W. and Cain, U. S. 1980. The children of teenage parents. *Fam. Plann. Perspect.* 12:34–43.
Bronfenbrenner, U. 1979. *The Ecology of Human Development.* Cambridge: Harvard University Press, Chapter 2.
Forbush, J. and Maciocha, T. 1981. Adolescent parent programs and family involvement. In T. Ooms (Ed.): *Teenage Pregnancy in a Family Context: Implications for Policy.* Philadelphia: Temple University Press.
Fox, G. 1981. The family's role in adolescent sexual behavior. In T. Ooms (Ed.): *Teenage Pregnancy in a Family Context: Implications for Policy.* Philadelphia: Temple University Press.

Furstenberg, F. F. 1976. *Unplanned Parenthood: The Social Consequences of Teenage Childbearing.* New York: Free Press.

Furstenberg, F. F. 1981. Implicating the family: teenage parenthood and kinship involvement. In T. Ooms (Ed.): *Teenage Pregnancy in a Family Context: Implications for Policy.* Philadelphia: Temple University Press.

Furstenberg, F. F., Herceg-Baron, R. and Jemail, J. 1981. Bringing in the family: kinship support and contraceptive behavior. In T. Ooms (Ed.): *Teenage Pregnancy in a Family Context: Implications for Policy.* Philadelphia: Temple University Press.

Gothard, S. 1980. The expanding right to treatment for minors: the legal implications for the enabling adults and disciplines. In M. Sugar (Ed.): *Responding to Adolescent Needs.* New York: Spectrum Publications.

Harper, J. 1981. *Assessing the Impact of Social Policies and Programs on Teenage Mothers and Their Families.* Final report of a Boston Family impact study. Available from the Family Impact Seminar, Suite 310, 1001 Connecticut Avenue, NW, Washington, DC 20036.

Hofmann, A. 1980. A rational policy toward consent and confidentiality in adolescent health care. *Adol. Health Care* 1:9–17.

Hofmann, A. D. and Moore, R. S. 1982. American Academy of Pediatrics Conference on Consent and Confidentiality in Adolescent Health Care. Washington, D.C.: American Academy of Pediatrics.

Minuchin, S. and Fishman, H. D. 1981. *Family Therapy Techniques.* Cambridge: Harvard University Press, Chapter 2.

Ooms, T. 1981. Introduction, and family involvement, notification, and responsibility: a personal essay. In T. Ooms (Ed.): *Teenage Pregnancy in a Family Context: Implications for Policy.* Philadelphia: Temple University Press.

Perlman, S. B. 1980. Pregnancy and parenting among runaway girls. *J. Fam. Issues* 1:202–273.

Pilpel, H. and Wechsler, N. 1971. Birth control, teenagers and the law. *Fam. Plann. Perspect.* 3:37–45.

Rosen, R. H. and Benson, T. 1979. *Help or Hindrance? Preliminary Findings on Pregnant Teenagers' Relations with Parents.* Presented at Annual Meeting of Society for Study of Social Problems, August.

Young, L. 1954. *Out of Wedlock: A Study of the Problems of the Unmarried Mother and Her Child.* New York: McGraw-Hill.

Index

Parity among adolescent mothers,
83-84
Pelvic inflammatory disease, 162
Planned Parenthood, 199, 205
Practicum sites for parenthood education, 151
Preeclampsia, 104
Pregnancy, adolescent
adult status from, 218
for avoidance of work, 30
class differences in handling of, 55
crises during, 103
crises precipitating, 25
decision-making in, 21-31
denial in, 25
Down's syndrome from, 103
drug and alcohol usage during, 104
economic deprivation with, 28
as escape from conflict, 24
ethnic factors in, 75-96
birth and delivery information,
84-85
contraceptive practices, 83
data base on, 77-85
economic situation, 77-78
educational history, 81-83
family background, 78-79
marital status, 79-81
parity, 83-84
prenatal history, 84-85
profile of black mother, 88-91
profile of hispanic mother,
91-95
extended family network with, 59
family context of, 215-224
male view of, 68
mental health programs for, 181-
193
community in, 182
description of, 185-188
in Hill Health Center, 183-185
in Parent-Infant Center, 188

[Pregnancy, adolescent]
[mental health programs for]
prevention of, 188-189
services of, 185
from misperception of risk, 160
mother-daughter symbiosis in, 56
narcissistic character disorders and,
24-25
in 19th century fiction, 3-20
oedipal issues in, 57, 60
oral dependency needs fulfilled by,
25
parental notification of, 211
poverty and, 25-26
prenatal care in, 59
preparation for, 141-154
characteristics of educational
programs on 151-154
child development programs on,
149-151
early programs on, 143-144
hospital and clinic programs on,
147-149
school programs on, 144-147
prevention programs for, 159, 191
as psychiatric disorder, 29, 60
psychodynamics of, 55-62, 190
psychological trauma of, 182
in response to loss, 25
risks and effects of, 102-106
self-concept in, 57
services for,
funding for, 192, 197-213
public sector management of,
198
settings for, 71-62
voluntarism in, 198
smoking during, 104
in South Africa, 101-102
statistics on, in US, 21, 101-102
syndrome of failure with, 25
tradition of, within families, 60